THE MYTH
OF PLANTAR
FASCIITIS

An Exploration of the Root Cause,
a Critical Review of Treatments,
and
the Importance of the EOTTS Solution!

MICHAEL E. GRAHAM,
DPM, FACFAS, FAENS, FAMIFAS, FACFAP

Published by Graham International Implant Institute
16137 Leone Drive
Macomb, MI 48042
www.Grahamiii.com

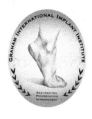

ISBN: 978-145757-044-5

This book is printed on acid-free paper.
Printed in the United States of America

ISBN
Digital edition published in 2019

Library of Congress Cataloging-in-Publication Data

Cover design by:

Printed and bound in the United States

The information in this book is for educational purposes only. It is not intended to replace the advice of a physician or medical practitioner.

This book is dedicated to the millions of people who suffer with **chronic** *heel pain and are searching for a better answer than to just "wait it out."*

Steps to Problem-Solving

Identify and Define the Problem

Analyze the Problem

Identify the Possible Solutions

Evaluate the Solutions

Select the Best Solution

Develop an Action Plan

Implement the Solution

Do not believe in anything simply because you have heard it.

Do not believe in anything simply because it is spoken and rumored by many.

But after observation and analysis, when you find that it agrees with reason, then accept it.

—Attributed to Buddha

Contents

Acknowledgments

Although heel pain is not a life-threatening illness, it has a significant impact on quality of life and on health in general. I have taken a step back for a new and critical look at the diagnosis and most commonly recommended treatments for it, spending many years researching medical journals for peer-reviewed evidence to substantiate the current theories and treatments. Along the way, I've discovered a major flaw in diagnosis—and, therefore, treatment—that is the reason most patients require a year or more to recover.

The valuable information provided by researchers needs greater attention and awareness. My goal is to present that information to you, the reader, with hope that if the underlying cause of your heel pain is adequately addressed (the sooner, the better), you can have a faster recovery.

I thank the global community of researchers who have taken the time to publish their findings.

Finally, thank you to my wife and daughter for allowing me to take time away from them to put my thoughts onto paper. Without their love and support, this book would not have been written.

Introduction

As many as three million adults limp in pain every time they stand up from sitting or lying down, or when they simply walk. Severe shooting pain can last from minutes to hours, depending on how long the pain has existed. The longer the pain has been occurring, the longer it will recur. Effective early treatment is key. As with any illness, the sooner a proper diagnosis is made and correct treatment begins, the more easily the pain or **symptoms** should go away.

Patients diagnosed with heel pain are typically told it will take a year or longer for the pain to go away. Advised to do stretching exercises and given pain pills or injections into their heel, these patients continue with life — in pain. Some patients are lucky enough to find some relief from those treatments, but the reality is that most patients will suffer many months of chronic pain. In the meantime, their quality of life and their health in general are negatively affected.

It's been estimated that nearly $400 million dollars a year is spent on treating heel pain![1] As a foot specialist, I have tried many different treatments over the years for heel pain, from very conservative to extreme (complicated **hindfoot** surgery). An internet search will reveal many options to bring relief — but do they work? No.

Why is **heel pain** so difficult to get rid of? What's really causing the problem? What if we've been focusing our attention in the wrong direction?

Now it's time for me to unveil the solution: EOTTS (extra-**osseous talotarsal** stabilization)! In this book, I will explain why chronic heel pain is often never cured, and what EOTTS is and why it works. You will come to understand why common treatments for chronic heel pain are designed to treat only the symptoms and to keep you in pain.

Imagine that your car isn't driving correctly. You take your car to the mechanic, and he says the problem is the steering. You pay a lot of money to get the steering realigned, but the problem still isn't fixed. Then you take your car to another mechanic, who says the axles are bent, so you get new axles. Still, your car is not driving correctly. You then go to the tire shop and have new tires put on your car, which works for a while, but after several months, the steering is off again. Why is this going on?

The problem is that no one has taken into consideration the *alignment of the tires*. Alignment of the base of any structure is very important. EOTTS is the alignment of *your structural base*! Keep that in mind as you read this book.

Moral of this story:
*If you don't know what's wrong,
you can't fix it.*

1

Fix the Cause, Not the Symptom

Each year, hundreds of millions of dollars are spent treating heel pain. The symptom—complex heel pain—is one of the most common yet downplayed and undercorrected foot complaints. A diagnosis of an "inflammatory condition" of the plantar fascia, a strong **ligament**-like **tissue** on the bottom of the foot, is made: **plantar fasciitis**. This book is focused on helping you understand the real cause of this grueling chronic foot pain and how it can be effectively addressed.

What causes this tissue to become dis-eased? The answer is *faulty foot mechanics*. When your **anklebone** and heel bone are not aligned correctly, the stability between these bones is lost, and you have a recipe for *pain*! For most patients with chronic foot pain, faulty foot mechanics are the missing link, often overlooked or undertreated. The ultimate problem is that the cause—that is, the etiology—of plantar fasciitis is not being treated. In fact, the cause is grossly ignored, overlooked, and undertreated. It seems that everything *except* the misalignment gets fixed! Doctors focus their attention in the wrong direction, treating the *symptoms*, rather than the *cause*. Why is this? Because they have been trained to treat the *symptoms*, despite the fact that their treatments fail miserably, over and over again.

In a typical scenario, a patient—let's call her Mrs. Jones—limps into Dr. Foot's office with a complaint of pain in her heel. After a foot exam, the doctor determines that Mrs. Jones has plantar fasciitis. The plantar fascia is the thick band of tissue on the bottom of the foot that supports the inner arch. The -*itis* means **inflammation**, even though it has been proven that the cells are *not* inflamed (more on that later)! So, problem #1: incorrect diagnosis of the cause of pain.

Then Dr. Foot explains Mrs. Jones's options for treatment. "Well, Mrs. Jones," he says, "we need to get you into a pair of custom arch supports/**orthotics** to start. Try that out for a bit. Also, I would like you to take these prescription anti-inflammatories."

Eight hundred dollars and two months later, Mrs. Jones returns to Dr. Foot's office with the same pain. "It has not gone away." She explains to the doctor, "The orthotics helped a little at first, but then my feet became as painful as before."

Dr. Foot now offers Mrs. Jones cortisone injections. He says she will "see a big improvement," so she gets three painful cortisone injections in the bottom of her inner heel. "Mrs. Jones, this will make you feel so much better," Dr. Foot assures her.

In just a few days, Mrs. Jones feels amazing. She is once again able to play tennis with her best friend—something she has avoided for months. "I can't believe it!" she tells her friend. "My foot pain is so much better!"

Mrs. Jones and her friend continue meeting frequently for tennis over several weeks until one morning, Mrs. Jones cannot stand when she tries to get out of bed. She cannot place her feet on the ground. The foot pain is back, and this time, with a vengeance!

Mrs. Jones is in tears. She thought everything was fixed! How could this have happened? Why did the pain come back?

Although Mrs. Jones had received some relief at first from the injections, the pain returned, worse than before, because the injections had only masked the pain and she had continued to be active, traumatizing the plantar fascia. Because the underlying problem did not get fixed, the symptoms were only temporarily masked.

Dr. Foot had X-rayed Mrs. Jones's foot on her first visit, but that was only to check if she had broken her heel bone or if a painful "spur" was present. That was the first problem. If Dr. Foot had examined the X-rays more closely, he could have made a very important finding that is usually missed: The alignment and stability of the anklebone on the heel bone were off. Had he noticed this, Dr. Foot likely could have diagnosed the faulty foot mechanics as the *actual* problem and would have been able to treat that instead of the symptom—plantar "fasciitis."

Without *all* the information, Dr. Foot will fail his patient, and Mrs. Jones will limp unhappily ever after, until possibly, the plantar fascia **ruptures** one day (*Ouch!*), or on the brighter side, she will come across this book and find the answer to her prayers.

Dr. Foot is not alone in directing the majority of his medical knowledge toward the plantar fascia. Our real concern, however, is his treatment for the underlying cause.

It is time for those doctors treating heel pain originating with biomechanical instability (that is, pain not due to things such as **trauma**, **bone tumors**, **stress fractures**, rheumatoid **arthritis**, and **sarcoidosis**) to realize that hindfoot instability is the root cause of heel pain. "So, Doc," you're probably asking, "what should the diagnosis be, if it's not plantar fasciitis?"

The cause of plantar fasciitis: hindfoot instability. A partially or fully obliterated (closed) **sinus tarsi** (the space between the heel bones) is the culprit! It is hindfoot instability that is the cause of plantar fasciitis, and plantar fasciitis is merely the result—the symptom—of that hindfoot instability!

"What? That sounds serious!" you might be saying. Well, while this problem can lead to tremendous, unbearable pain, surprisingly, there is a rather simple and easy solution to treat it. Simply put, if this naturally occurring space, the sinus tarsi, is closed or partially closed, the foot turns inward on every step taken. This results in extra motion and forces being placed on the **soft tissues**, muscles, ligaments, and bones of the foot, not to mention all the extra force traveling up the skeletal system to the knees, hip, back, and shoulders, eventually showing up as pain later. The entire musculoskeletal path is off-kilter as a result. So, to keep this space open and allow normal motion to take place while removing the excessive **pathology**-inducing motion, a **stent**—the HyProCure—is sized and simply pushed into place. Just as a cardiac-artery stent keeps the artery open to allow normal blood flow, this titanium stent keeps the sinus-tarsi **joint** space open to allow normal motion but also removes the excessive motion on the foot. Subsequently, the problem is solved! Finally, the healing cells can go to work to repair the years of damage that have been placed on the plantar fascia.

As we've already discussed, doctors need to go beyond the symptoms and treat the *cause*; otherwise, they are doing their patients a major disservice.

If you have a water leak in your basement, do you want to continuously mop up the water without ever fixing the problem, or do you want to find and then repair the leak?

Repair the leak, then mop the floor!

Studies have shown that if you correct the faulty alignment in a patient's foot, placing the foot back into its proper position, the **strain** and pressure on surrounding tissues will be relieved.[2-4] The only proven treatment that accomplishes this is EOTTS with *HyProCure*. EOTTS stands for extra-osseous talotarsal stabilization:

- **extra-osseous** (*extra-* means it does not involve bone (*osseous*));
- **talotarsal** (the joint in question that needs to be properly aligned); and
- **stabilization** (maintaining the correct position of the joint).

HyProCure is the stent implant that will accomplish this task.

EOTTS treatment does not involve any bone cutting or drilling. It is a soft-tissue procedure with a titanium stent, HyProCure (GraMedica, Macomb, Michigan), inserted into a naturally occurring space located between the ankle and heel bones. This procedure takes about fifteen minutes and can be performed under **twilight sedation**, a mild dose of general anesthesia, or just local anesthesia. The incision is less than one inch and is placed below and slightly in front of the outer anklebone.

Because it is classified as a minimally invasive soft-tissue procedure, EOTTS is the perfect choice for those doctors who are tired of the conservative treatments that just don't work but who run the opposite way when it comes to extreme rearfoot surgery. EOTTS is also the perfect choice for those patients who are tired of doctors who neglect to treat the *cause* of their chronic foot pain.

For peace of mind, it is important to understand that EOTTS is completely reversible. The stent can always be removed, but there is a less than 6 percent chance that it will need to be removed when placed into an ideal candidate's foot. This procedure is time-tested and evidence-based.

Patients are typically advised to exhaust all conservative treatment options and to wait months and months in the hope that their symptoms may gradually resolve, while never being told about EOTTS—just to avoid surgery This isn't major rearfoot surgery, however. (I would avoid that too!) It's a minimal-incision surgery that has *proven* clinical results (see references in the endnotes).

Although conservative treatments have helped a few lucky patients, most others will have continued pain, will experience a recurrence of pain, or worse, develop advanced secondary problems in their feet, knees, hips, or back. Some plantar fasciitis cases get to the point where the plantar fascia, that important band that supports the arch of the foot, ruptures, and then a cascade of issues tends to develop.

We can stop this from continuing! EOTTS is the solution, addressing chronic foot pain—plantar fasciitis—at its root, saving millions from lives of chronic foot pain.

Common treatments for heel pain that fail daily include taping, arch supports/foot orthotics, **night splints**, casting, physical therapy, lasers, **platelet-rich plasma** (PRP), cortisone injections, and shockwave therapy. How are these treatments supposed to put the foot back into alignment? They aren't. They are designed only to be supportive, to relieve symptoms—but in the meantime, the problem still exists and is worsening, because these treatments only address the symptoms!

The beauty of EOTTS with *HyProCure* is that it is a conservative internal option as the move away from invasive, traditional heel surgery for recurring or chronic heel pain. This treatment continues to grow in popularity, due to scientific studies showing detrimental effects from invasive heel surgery in which outer foot pain, decreased arch stability, and increased pain to the ball of the foot have been cited as complications.[5–7]

In comparison, most patients can walk, though in a limited capacity, immediately following the EOTTS procedure. Their faulty foot mechanics have been instantly and internally corrected, which prevents the advancement of other foot issues. Conversely, in radical rearfoot surgery, patients are off their feet for months, which usually contributes to advancing foot problems, and yet, the problem fails to be corrected! Why choose to have a radical surgical heel procedure that is *known* to cause other foot problems and has only a 65 percent long-term favorability?

It is appalling that the root cause of these diseases is not being addressed. It all boils down to alignment of your feet. Remember the example earlier about the alignment of your car? Consider hindfoot stability *your* proper alignment. Excessive motion in the foot not only contributes to heel pain but can also lead to **pathological** foot deformities such as **bunions**, **hammertoes**, blisters, corns, **calluses**, **heel spurs**, ingrown toenails, and others! This is well-documented.[8–10] Instead of concentrating on the symptoms of heel pain, the move toward stabilization of the hindfoot through EOTTS with sinus tarsi *HyProCure* stents has been found to be a reliable and cost-effective treatment option for chronic heel pain and is less invasive than typical rearfoot surgery. The EOTTS procedure treats hindfoot instability by realigning and stabilizing the anklebone. By doing so, it treats the *cause*, **not** the *symptoms*.

Facts, Figures, and Why You Should Care

First, I want to apologize for this chapter. It is somewhat dry reading, but I felt that it was important to include. It illustrates how common heel pain is and the consequences that ensue because of inappropriate treatment—by treating the *symptom*, rather than the *cause* of heel pain.

The number of patients going to their medical doctors to get a consultation from a foot specialist has increased over the past several years and continues to increase year after year, yet the cause of the problem keeps getting overlooked and left untreated, because the focus is on the *symptom*.

As many as three million Americans suffer with chronic pain to their inner heel every year.[11] That is a lot of people suffering from something that can be managed by simply solving the root of the problem. Imagine all the drugs pumped out of pharmacies that these people—people like you—are refilling each month—and the billions of dollars in revenue for pharmaceutical companies.

Health finance experts have also estimated that as much as $376 million a year is spent on doctor visits to treat this chronic pain.[12] While it's not the hundreds of billions of dollars spent treating heart disease and strokes, or the $157 billion spent on cancer care, it still is a significant amount of money. And we haven't even talked about lost wages from missed work because of heel pain!

Heel pain affects up to 10 percent of the population.[13] Most people with chronic heel pain are forty years and older. Many young professional athletes, however, have had their careers cut short by the chronic pain in their heels. Even worse, a high rate of **comorbidity** is associated with chronic heel pain, largely due to decreased activity. You aren't able to do the kinds of activities you'd like, because of the pain you suffer after being active. (This is called **activity-limiting pain**.)

If it hurts when you stand or walk, you quickly decrease the amount of walking or standing you do. Maybe your doctor instructed you during your last yearly checkup to walk and be active because you had some unexpected holiday weight gain, but when you follow his or her instructions, you are rewarded with excruciating pain to the bottom of your foot that makes your eyes bulge out. (Thanks, Doc!) So, you stop. Why do something that's going to cause you pain?

Decreased activity levels will lead to decreased metabolism. That means you'll start gaining weight. Maybe you're even rewarded with an extra ten pounds of fabulous belly-warming companionship, just in time for your niece Alyssa's wedding in June!

Decreased metabolism and weight gain can lead to obesity, and obesity leads to *all* sorts of medical conditions, such as high blood pressure, strokes, diabetes, heart disease, gallbladder disease, osteoarthritis, and even certain forms of cancer.[14,15] The list goes on, but I won't bore you. The leading recommendation for improving those diseases is to get out and walk and increase your metabolism. That's all good if your feet are in proper alignment (most people's aren't), but how are you supposed to know if your feet are aligned or not?

If you can't walk, you can't exercise, so those diseases don't get better; they get worse! Soon, not only do you have badly aching feet, but you are also taking pills for high blood pressure, along with insulin for your diabetes.

Eleven to fifteen percent of people who seek treatment from podiatric physicians present with heel pain as their main concern.[16] They have tried many other remedies and solutions, but unfortunately, they haven't gotten better. As we know from an earlier discussion, the sooner a medical problem is treated, the better. If you wait too long, more damage can occur, and it will take longer to treat and will be more difficult to fix, with more complex treatments, surgery, or medications.

Foot specialists often refer to heel pain as being self-limiting. When something is described as self-limiting, it means that the thing will go away completely and permanently *at some point*. (What's that supposed to mean? Oh, I know! This means "Actually, Patient, I really don't want to deal with this right now.")

It has often been said that the average time one should expect heel pain to last is about a year and a half. *A year and a half!* Even the motivated individual who is willing to suffer by waiting that out—taking the chance that the pain won't get worse and hoping that it actually will be self-limiting soon—must consider this: Even when heel pain seems to have gone away, its cause has *not*, and other conditions will surface thereafter.

Researchers have found that the average treatment of chronic heel pain is twelve months or longer, depending on the severity of the condition, how much damage is done, and of course, the types of treatments prescribed.[17] Conservative care, such as ice, stretching, rest, and/or night splints, has shown a wide range of "success," but 20 to 30 percent of patients progress to having a chronic condition.[18,19] The treatment and recovery for these patients who develop chronic conditions will be less predictable, more involved, and lengthier—and recurrence of pain will be common.

Besides causing or worsening the general health issues described earlier, heel pain can also alter the way you stand and walk. This "not normal" way of walking can have a negative effect on your knees, hips, and back. The last thing you want is to go from bad to worse, so let's *fix* the cause!

3

The Plantar Fascia and the Search for Truth

The fascia (*fah-she-ah*) is a specialized and extremely strong, soft connecting tissue. This kind of tissue is located in other areas of the body, too, but the thickest and strongest fibers are located on the bottom of the foot. Here, they are called plantar fascia. *Plantar* is the medical word for the bottom of the foot (just like plantar warts are warts on the bottom of your foot). The strong fibers attach the bottom of the heel bone to the ball of the foot. These fibers terminate into the joints where the toes attach to the foot.[20] The plantar-fascia tissue is firmly connected to both the skin on the bottom of the foot and to the muscles within the arch and the bottom of the foot (see figure 1).[21]

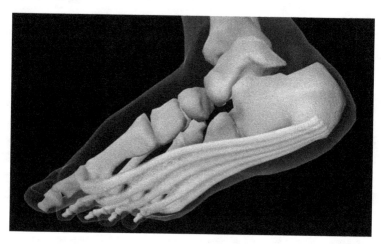

Figure 1. The plantar fascia is a broad band of tissue that connects the heel to the base of the toe bones.

This fascial tissue is different from **tendons**, which connect muscle to bone, and ligaments, which connect bone to bone. The strong collagen fibers of the fascia are arranged in multiple layers. The bundles of these fibers tend to be arranged at a 90-degree angle to those in the neighboring layers.

There are nerve sensors located within the tough fibers of the plantar fascia. In an extensive anatomical and **histologic** view (looking at the tissue under the microscope), Stecco et al. found that there are pressure sensors throughout the plantar fascia.[22] Another important finding is the presence of hyaluronan in the plantar fascia. This is a substance thought to be produced by the fasciacytes, which help to heal the damaged fascia.

Functions of the Plantar Fascia

The plantar fascia is important for foot function because it helps stabilize the inner arch of the foot.[23-25] The plantar fascia helps to transfer forces from the heel to the **forefoot** during the walking (**gait**) cycle.[26] Less well-known, but also a very important function of the plantar fascia, is its role in determining the position of the foot and controlling the muscles of the foot and lower leg.

When the heel touches the ground when walking, the plantar fascia is in a relaxed state. Later, when the heel starts to lift, the plantar fascia increases in length until the forefoot leaves the ground.[27] This is very important to understand, especially if there is excessive strain acting on the plantar fascia—as when the heel stays on the ground longer than it should during the walking cycle.

Chronic Heel Pain and the Inner Band of Plantar Fascia

Two main sections of the plantar fascia stabilize the inner and outer columns of the foot bones. The inner band of the plantar fascia supports the inner arch and has more strain acting on it than the outer band does. This is why the inner band is the thickest and broadest portion of the plantar fascia[28,29] and is also most commonly involved with chronic heel pain.

Research has shown that up to 1.5 times the body weight acts on the plantar fascia.[30–32] Maximum strain occurs to the innermost section of the fascia, and the least amount of strain occurs to the portion on the outer bottom side of the foot. A study by Chen et. al showed that patients with chronic heel pain in only the heel have increased fascia thickness and greater **vascularity** (i.e., blood vessel activity) on the affected side—the body's way of trying to heal the damaged fascia.[33]

There are many reasons someone could develop pain to the bottom of the heel. The majority of cases are common and clear-cut, but several factors must be considered in *all* cases. Most people in this modern age will consult with Dr. Internet prior to seeking a consultation from a medical professional. There is a lot of good information online, but also a lot of bad information that can be misleading and could delay the treatment of this condition, so a professional should always be consulted.

Unfortunately, misinformation also exists within the medical profession. I don't mean that your doctor visits the internet for advice on how to treat your condition, but if you've seen a doctor for your heel pain and your pain has not been relieved, then your doctor probably doesn't know about the simple solution discussed previously: EOTTS. Again, as we've already mentioned, most foot-care specialists are familiar with conservative, mostly temporary, treatments or with the off-the-chart "we're going to cut important tissues" treatments. I don't think doctors are completely to blame, because most medical schools also don't know of the solution for heel pain and, therefore, can't teach it. Doctors are *partially* to blame, though, because once they do get that degree, it's up to them to stay current on information and advances in medicine. Many, however, are close-minded.

The goal of treatment must be to identify and fix any underlying cause or problem.[34] Imagine you have an ingrown toenail. This also can be a very painful chronic condition, and it also has many forms of treatment, such as soaking your toe, wearing a cut-out or open-toe shoe, taking antibiotic pills, applying an antibiotic to the nail, taking pain pills, and whatever else you can think of. But for some reason, the pain just won't go away with these treatments. Why? Because they treat only the symptoms. The toenail is still digging into the skin of the toe, and the pain and symptoms will continue until that ingrown nail is removed from the skin.

We don't want to make the same mistakes with diagnosing and treating your chronic heel pain by addressing only the symptoms. Patients who are overweight, have had chronic pain in both heels, and have had symptoms for a prolonged period are going to take a lot longer to get better. That's why it's so important for you to seek medical care from a qualified foot specialist right away.[35]

It's therefore up to *you*, the patient, to get informed and get an exact diagnosis and information about your options. And yes, once you have finished this book, you probably will know more about this condition than most medical professionals out there.

4

Twenty Important Questions

This chapter offers a brief explanation of the importance of these questions to aid your doctor in discovering why you have heel pain. Sometimes, the doctor may assume they know what's wrong, but a valuable piece of information, such as your answer to one of these questions, could provide a clearer path to a more appropriate diagnosis.

We have briefly discussed that the main reason for heel pain is the misalignment of the foot bones, which "closes" the **sinus tarsi**, the naturally occurring space between the ankle and heel bones. Other things can also contribute to heel pain, however. These less-common causes of heel pain can include **fracture** of the heel bone, bone tumors /cysts, and arthritis conditions (rheumatoid, gout, psoriatic, trauma, and lupus).

Specific questions and information about specific symptoms will help in the diagnostic process, as they help us rule in or **rule out** the less common causes of heel pain. During the clinical examination, a practitioner will ask questions about your medical history and questions directed to the nature of the pain (sharp, dull), when the pain occurs, where specifically it occurs, if it spreads, what makes it worse, and what makes it better. Specific key clinical and **radiographic** findings will additionally help the foot-care specialist diagnose the problem.

Now let's walk through a proper exam.

There are three parts to a proper foot exam, allowing the physician to make a diagnosis and advise you about proper treatment: questions about your medical history and current symptoms, a physical exam, and a radiographic exam. We will discuss each part in some detail in this book, but this chapter is focused on the questions section. The physical and radiographic exams will be discussed in subsequent chapters.

Continuing with our example of Mrs. Jones, we're going to examine how her first visit to Dr. Foot *should* have gone, beginning with the questions he should have asked, along with some reasons for why these questions are helpful.

Questions

1. **Mrs. Jones, have you had similar heel pain previously?**

   If you've had this problem before, in one or both heels, this will also be valuable for the doctor to know because it's easier to get rid of the heel pain the first time. The second time is more difficult because there will be *scar tissue* from the first bout; scar tissue makes treating the pain more difficult.

2. **Mrs. Jones, where *specifically* does your heel hurt? Where is the bull's-eye, the center of the pain?**

   The location of the **center point of pain** (figure 2) will help determine the *underlying issue*.

   - Pain to the **inner side, not the bottom of the heel,** is usually caused by a nerve **entrapment**.
   - Pain in the **arch** could be caused by a variety of issues.
   - Pain to the **bottom inner heel** suggests partially damaged plantar fascia tissue.

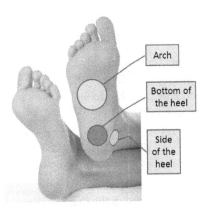

Figure 2. There are two different locations where the plantar fascia fibers become damaged. This book focuses on the bottom inner heel area.

3. Mrs. Jones, do you have pain in both heels? Or just one?

   Unfortunately, the longer you have pain in one heel, the *more likely* you are to develop it in both, so it's important to know if we're dealing with one or both feet.

4. Mrs. Jones, *how long* has this been present?

   - The longer the pain has been present, the more tissue damage could be involved.
   - Pain or symptoms that have been occurring less than three months are usually considered **acute**, and conservative care will be more effective.
   - Pain for more than three months is considered a **chronic** condition, and conservative care will be *less* effective.

5. Mrs. Jones, *when*, specifically, does your heel hurt?

   - If your heel hurts *all the time*, whether you are sitting or standing, that points to certain causes.
   - Does your heel hurt only when you *first get up to walk in the morning*, but not the rest of the day?
   - If your heel is painful *without easing up*, that is an indication of a more serious condition than plantar fascial disease.

6. Mrs. Jones, how long does it hurt?

   This is connected to the question of when the pain is experienced and gives clues about how much tissue damage there is.

   - Is the pain present for only a few seconds or minutes when you get on your feet?
   - Do you have pain that doesn't go away and is constant whenever you're walking?

7. Mrs. Jones, does it go away with more walking?

   Some patients relate that the pain is only in their heel for a short time in the morning with the first few steps, but after they walk for a while, it eases up or completely disappears, only to reappear the next morning.

This information provides clues to the severity of the plantar-fascia tissue damage. The longer it takes for the pain to subside, the greater the tissue damage. The more quickly the pain resolves, the less tissue damage is present.

8. **Mrs. Jones, does the pain get worse with more walking?**

   Whether the pain goes away with walking or gets worse with walking leads to different diagnoses.

9. **Mrs. Jones, do you have burning in your heel?**

   The *type* of pain felt is connected to the location of the pain and can also help determine the underlying issue.

   Burning pain usually involves a **nerve**.

10. **Mrs. Jones, does it feel like a needle or thumbtack is stabbing into your inner heel?**

    Stabbing or **shooting pain**, like burning pain, is also usually associated with nerve involvement but can lead to different diagnoses.

11. **Mrs. Jones, does the pain extend into the arch of your foot or up the inner heel?**

    It is very important to diagnosis for the examiner to know whether the pain is localized (i.e., pinpointed to one area) or spreads out to other areas of the foot.

12. **Mrs. Jones, what makes your foot feel better?**

    This question seems somewhat silly, but it is very important.

    - Does it feel better when you're *on* your foot or *off* your foot?
    - Does ice help?
    - Have you taken any over-the-counter or prescription pills that have been beneficial?
    - Have different shoes helped? What about stopping exercise? Elevating your feet?

13. **What makes it feel worse?**

    - Does ice make it hurt more? Does it hurt when you're walking or running?
    - Have you noticed that the longer you are on your feet, the more you suffer after?

14. **What have you tried to make it better?**

    This is important for your doctor to know, because if you've already tried something, there's no use in trying it again.

    Many home remedies exist—rolling your heel on a golf or tennis ball, icing your heel, soaking your feet in hot water or **Epsom salt**, and over-the-counter heel cups, arch supports, or night splints—but are they working?

15. **How active were you prior to developing this heel pain?**

    The reason for asking this question is to correlate an increase in **weightbearing**/walking activity, which increases the strain on the plantar fascia.

    - Most adults who develop heel pain don't recall any trauma causing it. They were very active and just woke up one morning with heel pain.
    - Many led active lifestyles and exercised, and walking did not lead to any pain; others did more walking or standing than usual (over a weekend, for instance) and then woke up the next day with heel pain.

16. **Mrs. Jones, what type of work do you perform? Do you stand or walk for your job?**

    People who stand or walk for a living will take longer to "heal" than people who have sedentary jobs.

17. **What kind of exercises did you perform? Walking, treadmill, running?**

    This goes back to the *activity level prior to developing heel pain.* Typically, more active people will develop heel pain than those who are less active.

18. **What kind of shoes do you wear?**

    Believe it or not, people who wear a slight heel—about two inches—are *less* likely to develop heel pain than people who wear flats. That's because the elevated heel on the shoe helps decrease the strain on the tissue on the bottom of the foot.

    A situation can arise in which someone who normally wears a heel and then does a lot of walking in flats develops heel pain. This is because the tissues of their feet have slightly contracted because they aren't being stretched out with heels, and wearing flats causes an overstretching of the tissues.

19. How often do you change your shoes?

The type of shoes worn regularly or semi-regularly affects the strain placed on the tissues on the bottom of the foot. Worn-out shoes alter the way you walk and lead to overstretching of the tissues on the bottom of your foot.

Even worse, most wear their old beat-up shoes to do yard work over the weekend. When Monday morning comes along, so does the heel pain! It's no surprise that Mondays get a bad rap.

20. Mrs. Jones, have you gone to other medical professionals for help?

This is a similar and important question to the self-remedies that you've tried. If you've been examined and treated by another medical professional, your current practitioner is going to want to know what they tried. Again, we don't want to try something that didn't work.

- Did they give you injections or other treatments?
- What helped? What made it better?
- What made it worse?

Now that we've covered the questions you need to be prepared to answer when you see a doctor about your heel pain, let's discuss the other things a doctor worth his or her salt is going to do if you come in complaining of heel pain.

5

Physical Examination of Your Feet

This second part of the exam consists of two separate aspects—sitting (**non-weightbearing**) and standing (weightbearing)—to assess joint stability and alignment. We'll look at each in detail in this chapter.

Sitting (Non-Weightbearing) Exam

Practitioners need to examine the stability and the **range of motion** of the joints in the foot and ankle. This part of the examination is why we foot specialists exist. A physician must be able to *think beyond* the obvious to come to an accurate diagnosis and treatment for the patient. Most medical professionals can check if a pulse is present, push on someone's foot to determine where the pain is located, or spot a callus on the bottom of a foot, but the joint portion of the exam is the most difficult. One joint is often understated, even in orthopedics, and warrants more attention: the *talotarsal joint.*

The talotarsal joint is the most important joint of the foot. It is the "foundation" joint, in addition to being one of the most complicated joints of the body. It is formed by the **talus** (anklebone), the **calcaneus** (heel bone), and the **navicular** (bone in front of the anklebone). In between the ankle and heel bones is a naturally occurring space called the sinus tarsi (figure 3).

There is a reason this joint is so important: *The entire weight of the body rests on it.* Additionally, the complex motions between the ankle and hindfoot bones are responsible for the **locking** (**supination**) and unlocking (**pronation**) of the bones of the foot.

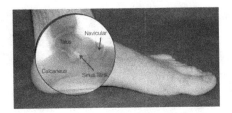

Figure 3. X-ray overlay showing normal alignment of the hindfoot bones.

The motions of *supination* and *pronation* begin and end with the motion of the anklebone on the hindfoot bones. It is very important for you to understand the difference between these two motions, *pronation* and *supination*, as we work our way to a true cause of your heel pain.

Supination motion *locks*, or *stabilizes*, the joints and is more important than pronation. Pronation is the opposite motion, *unlocking* the joints of the foot and making the joints within the foot *unstable*.

We need to have a slight amount of pronation. When the foot first touches the ground or another weightbearing surface, the pronation motion allows the foot to become a **mobile adapter**. In other words, it allows the foot to compensate when you walk on uneven ground.

It is important to determine the amount of supination or pronation occurring within the foundation joint, because too much pronation leads to many foot and ankle disorders. A qualified foot doctor evaluates this by applying pressure under the outer part of the foot, just behind the fourth and fifth toes—specifically, under the **anatomic necks** of the fourth and fifth metatarsal bones—pushing this part of the foot upward and outward (see figure 4).

A stable joint will have only a few degrees of motion, but an unstable foot will have more than a few degrees of motion.

A normal foot will have two-thirds supination but only one-third pronation.

Of course, other parts of the foot must be checked as well. For instance, the first metatarsal bone should be checked for stability. The first metatarsal is the long bone behind the big toe. Normally, this bone should be stable and the examiner should detect only minimal motion in it.

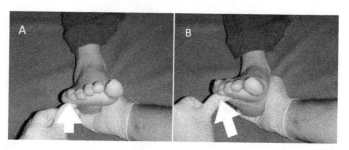

Figure 4. To test the stability of the hindfoot bones, maximum force is applied to the outer part of the foot. (A) shows the normal amount of pronation, just a few degrees of motion. (B) shows excessive motion, > 6 degrees, which indicates excessive pronation.

Another part of the foot to be checked is the big-toe joint. There should be plenty of motion here; limited motion will alter the way you walk.

Finally, the doctor should evaluate the range of motion of your ankle joint. Limited ankle-joint motion could be a contributing factor to heel pain. Specifically, a tight Achilles tendon is also known to be associated with heel pain.

Now that we've made it through the sitting part of the exam, let's look at the standing exam.

Standing (Weightbearing) Exam

This is another part of the exam that most medical professionals skip or overlook. You need to get off the exam table, stand, and walk. Most patients have more pain either *while* standing or walking or *after* they have stood or walked, so walking and standing probably have something to do with why you have pain in your heel. Failure to examine the alignment and stability of your feet when you are standing and walking will prevent the examiner from determining the real cause of your heel pain. Let's discuss some of the things a thorough weight-bearing exam will be looking at.

Lower-Leg Alignment

A first consideration is to simply look at the alignment of the lower leg with the forefoot. Normally, the leg should **line up** with the foot (figure 5). If the foot turns outward, this is a clue that there is an alignment issue between the leg and foot.

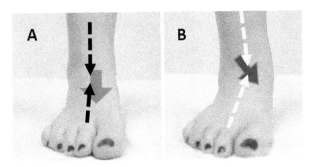

Figure 5. (A) Stable hindfoot alignment. (B) Abnormal hindfoot-to-forefoot alignment.

Inner Arch

The inner arch area should be looked at after weight has been applied to the foot. The arch should basically stay the same and shouldn't lower when you are standing (figure 6). A *lowered* or *flat arch* is also an indication of an alignment issue.

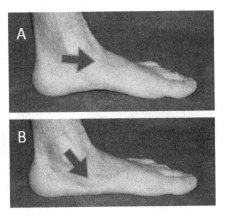

Figure 6. (A) Aligned hindfoot and naturally appearing arch. (B) Lowered arch resulting from misaligned hindfoot bones, which increases the strain to the plantar fascia.

Back-of-Heel Alignment (Too Many Toes?)

Finally, a look at the back of the heel is necessary. The heel should line up with the lower leg. Many people with chronic heel pain have heels that turn outward (figure 7).

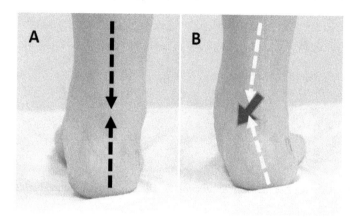

Figure 7. (A) Aligned hindfoot. (B) Outward curvature of the heel bone resulting from misaligned hindfoot bones.

While looking at the back of the foot, the skilled foot doctor also looks to see if you have "too many toes" visible. Normally, only the fifth and maybe a small portion of the fourth toe should be visible. If more than the fifth and fourth toes are visible, you have "too many toes." This also means you have a foot-alignment issue.

Walk

The skilled doctor will have you walk a bit so he or she can look at the backs of your ankles and feet. Again, the doctor is looking for the turning out of the heel and "too many toes," which may not appear when you are standing but *will* appear when you're walking.

By the end of the physical exam, the doctor will have observed any orthopedic conditions (faulty foot mechanics) that could have led to strain on your plantar-fascia tissue. At this point, the doctor will want to look at the bone alignment with the use of X-rays or **ultrasonic imaging**, which will be discussed in the next two chapters.

Developing Your X-ray Vision

The final part of your examination for foot pain should be X-rays of your feet. The *only* way a doctor can make a proper and accurate diagnosis of your foot condition is to use, in combination with the physical examination, X-rays of your feet taken while you are *standing* (weightbearing).

Let me say that again: The *only* way a doctor can make a *proper* and *accurate* diagnosis of your foot condition is to use, in combination with the physical examination, X-rays of your feet taken while you are standing.

X-rays taken when you are *not* standing are basically useless! Yes, useless! Although they can determine in this case if you have a broken bone, they cannot accurately determine the *misalignment* of your foot.

If your foot doctor orders X-rays in the non-standing, non-weightbearing position, a red flag should be set in your mind. You know enough right now from what we have discussed so far to question it. You know that the talotarsal joints are the foundation of the body and carry the body's weight, so if you are *not* in a weightbearing stance, the X-ray can produce a false negative, and the problem will go undiagnosed.

Within this standing position, two different standing stances need to be X-rayed for each foot: *relaxed stance* and *neutral stance*.

For each of these stances (relaxed and neutral), two radiographic views need to be taken per foot: *lateral* (side) view and *dorsoplantar* (front). The first set of X-rays is taken when you are simply standing in a normal fashion, as you would at any time. The second set of X-rays is taken after your foot has been guided into its correct position, or its ideal alignment, by the doctor or X-ray technician (figure 8). This means that each foot will require four total X-rays:

a. Relaxed stance (lateral)

b. Neutral (corrected) stance (lateral)

c. Relaxed stance (dorsoplantar)

d. Neutral (corrected) stance (dorsoplantar)

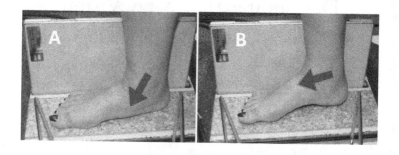

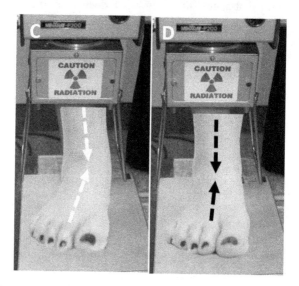

Figure 8. Foot position for comparison X-ray views (A) Relaxed-stance (misaligned). (B) Foot in corrected stance (aligned).

After the X-rays are taken, the doctor will gather information from them to reinforce and confirm what he or she learned by rounding up information in the question phase and narrowing down the possibilities during the physical phase of the exam. Information from all parts of the exam is thus used by the doctor to reach a diagnosis, with the properly taken X-rays undoubtedly confirming it.

Now it's time to learn how to read your X-rays so you can see what the doctor sees. This is not going to make you an expert, but the more you know, the better choice you have to make the most fitting and appropriate treatment for your chronic heel pain.

The Lateral (Side) View X-ray

Remember, the lateral view X-ray is taken in a standing relaxed stance and in a standing neutral stance.

- The doctor will be looking at these things:
- Bone fractures or tumors
- Sinus tarsi space
- Anklebone alignment
- Heel bone alignment
- **Cyma line** (compares the end of the anklebone with the end of the heel bone)
- Navicular bone position
- Arthritis
- First metatarsal stability
- Big-toe joint

Fracture or Other Abnormal Finding

We want to see if there is a heel-bone fracture or other abnormal bone finding in the area where you are experiencing pain. Many types of bone and other soft-tissue problems can also cause heel pain.

Because of how much heel pain has been blamed on heel spurs, the area where spurs occur is also one of the first areas of the heel that we look at in X-rays. (Chapter 11 is devoted to heel spurs, so we're not going into detail about them here.)

Sinus Tarsi

The sinus tarsi and the alignment of the ankle and heel bones are of importance in the diagnosis of anklebone instability and misalignment of the foot as the cause of heel pain. These are especially important and relevant to misaligned feet. Remember, the sinus tarsi should be *open*. If the sinus tarsi is closed or narrowed, we have an anklebone instability issue. There aren't any specific degrees or measurements for the opening of the sinus tarsi space, because everyone's space will look a little different, but it's very easy to see whether the space is open or closed (figure 9).

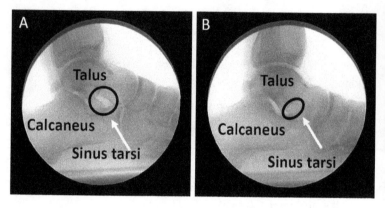

Figure 9. X-ray of the sinus tarsi: open, normal (left) and closed, abnormal (right).

Talus (Anklebone) Alignment

Next, the doctor bisects the anklebone in the lateral X-ray, drawing a line to divide the upper and lower sections of anklebone, as shown in figure 10. (Most times, the doctor will do this mentally, rather than drawing it on the X-ray.) That line should extend into the long first metatarsal bone of the forefoot (see figure). If the anklebone **bisection** falls *below the first metatarsal bone,* this is an indication that there is an *anklebone alignment issue* (figure 10, photo A).

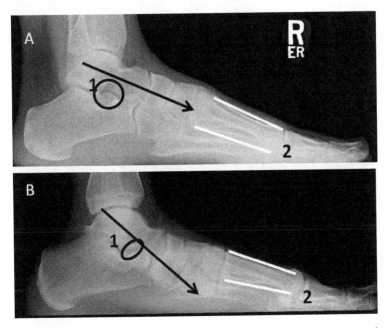

Figure 10. (A) Bisection of the talus (1) extending into the area of the first metatarsal bone indicated by the two white lines (2). (B) Bisection of the talus (1) that does not extend into the first metatarsal bone (2) due to the partial dislocation of the talus.

Calcaneal Inclination Angle (Heel Bone Alignment)

The next area viewed on the lateral view X-ray should be the angle between the bottom of the heel bone and the bottom of the foot. This is called the **calcaneal inclination angle**. Normally, the heel bone should be angulated 21 degrees from the bottom of the foot (figure 11, photo A). Many patients with chronic heel pain, however, will have a calcaneal inclination angle less than 21 degrees (figure 11, photo B).

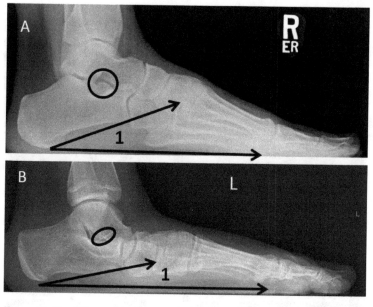

Figure 11. The calcaneus inclination angle formed by the bottom of the foot and bottom border of the heel bone: normal angle (A) and lower-than-normal angle (B).

Cyma Line

The **cyma line** is a lesser known but also very important finding. ("Cyma" means "curvy line.") The cyma line occurs at the front of the ankle and heel bones. Normally, the head of the anklebone should be just barely in front of the heel bone (figure 12, photo A). When the anklebone has a stability issue, it will slide forward more than it is supposed to when standing (figure 12, photo B). This will then increase the strain to the tissues on the inner and bottom parts of the foot. This landmark finding of cyma line advancement can occur only with the associated pathologic closure of the sinus tarsi.

The best way to see the difference in alignment is with the comparison X-rays, which is why it is important to take X-ray views in both the relaxed and neutral stances (figure 12) of the anklebone.

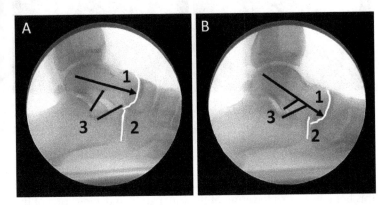

Figure 12. (A) Aligned hindfoot: (1) head of the anklebone, (2) front end of the heel bone, and (3) boundaries of the open sinus tarsi. (B) The anklebone has partially displaced on the heel bone; the head of the anklebone (1) has pushed forward in relation to the front of the heel bone (2), and the sinus tarsi has narrowed. This increases the strain on the plantar fascia.

Navicular Bone Stability

The navicular is the bone in front of the anklebone, and its position should be evaluated when looking for the cause of heel pain. Just like for the sinus tarsi, there are no specific measurements to distinguish between normal (figure 13, photo A) and abnormal (figure 13, photo B) navicular positioning. When seen on the lateral-view X-ray, the bottom of the navicular bone should be located above the midway line of the cuboid bone—the bone in front of the heel bone.

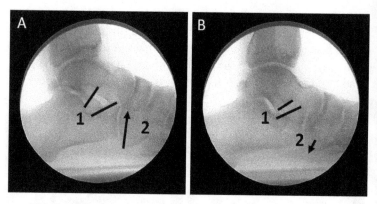

Figure 13. (A) The anklebone aligned on the heel bone. The sinus tarsi is open (1) and the navicular bone is aligned (2). (B) Partial dislocation of the anklebone closing the sinus tarsi (1), forcing the navicular bone to sag or drop (2).

The position of the navicular is important because the lowering of this bone leads to a lowering of the inner arch, and a lowering of the inner arch increases the strain to the tissues on the inner bottom of the foot (i.e., plantar fascia).

Midfoot Arthritis

Depending on your age, you could develop arthritis in the **midfoot**, the result of decades of excessive forces acting on the joints and soft tissue. Arthritis is taken into consideration because of the types of treatments that are available. If little to no arthritis is seen, more treatments are available. Severe arthritis (figure 14) will limit treatment options, which is why it's better to seek medical attention sooner than later when you begin to experience foot pain.

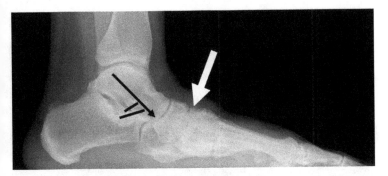

Figure 14. Decades of walking on a partially dislocating anklebone has led to micro-trauma to the midfoot joints. The chronic inflammatory reaction leads to arthritic disease in the midfoot (white arrow).

Stability of the First Metatarsal Bone

The longest bone in the forefoot is the first metatarsal bone. The alignment of this bone with the anklebone must be taken into consideration when looking at the causes of heel pain. When we walk, the majority of the pressure from the body's weight passes through—or at least is *supposed* to pass through—the end of the first metatarsal bone (figure 15, photo A).

Instability of the hindfoot causes the weight to fall differently, however, thus increasing the forces acting on the end of the first metatarsal bone. This, in turn, can lead to weakness at the joint with the midfoot, causing an abnormal elevation of the first metatarsal bone, which means there will be increased forces acting on the inner soft tissues on the bottom of the foot (figure 15, photo B).

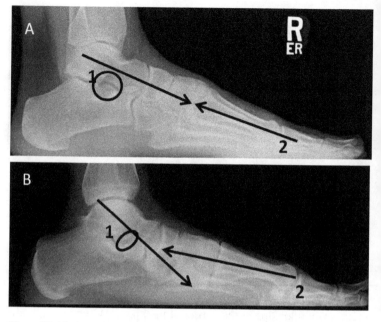

Figure 15. (A) An open sinus tarsi with an aligned and stable anklebone. The bisection of the anklebone (1) lines up with the first metatarsal bone (2). (B) Abnormal closure of the sinus, indicating a partial dislocation of the ankle bone. The bisection of the ankle bone (1) falls below the bisection of the first metatarsal bone (2).

Big-Toe Joint

One of the last areas to look at is the big-toe joint. Many patients with chronic heel pain have limited or even no motion here. As we said just above, the weight of the body—at least most of it—passes through the first metatarsal bone, which ends at the big-toe joint. Limited motion in the big-toe joint will force the forefoot to turn outward, which will also lead to increased strain to the inner arch of the foot (figure 16).

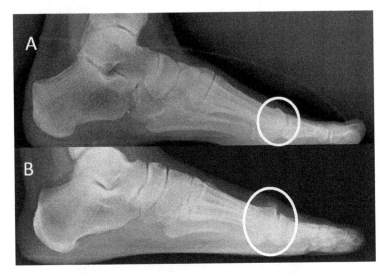

Figure 16. (A) Normal, healthy big-toe joint. (B) Large bone spur formation on the top of the big-toe joint from years of excessive forces from excessive hindfoot motion.

Now let's focus our attention on the other important X-ray view of the foot. This is the top-to-bottom view, medically called the dorso-plantar, or DP, view.

Dorsoplantar View X-ray

The DP view of the foot X-ray is used to determine if other findings are present that could be factors in the development or cause of heel pain. Again, any obvious fracture or tumors will be looked for, but the main focus is the alignment of the anklebone with other bones of the foot, especially the forefoot.

Hindfoot-to-Forefoot Alignment

A very quick and easy way to determine the alignment between the anklebone and forefoot is to draw a bisection of the anklebone. A normal alignment should find the bisection of the anklebone within the first metatarsal bone or even in the space between the first and second metatarsal bones (figure 17, photo A). An abnormal alignment can be assumed if the bisection falls inward of the first metatarsal bone (figure 17, photo B).

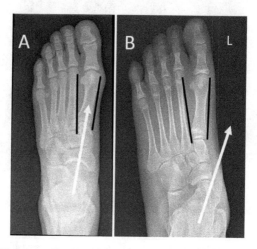

Figure 17. (A) A normally aligned hindfoot to forefoot. (B) A partially displaced anklebone; the bisection of the anklebone has turned inward and no longer falls between the black lines.

An angular measurement between the bisection of the ankle and second metatarsal bone should be made. Unfortunately, many medical professionals will compare the anklebone alignment with the first metatarsal bone. We don't want to use that measurement alone, however, because many people also have an abnormal deviation of the first metatarsal bone, where the first metatarsal bone moves away from the second metatarsal bone. Measuring an angle between two deviated bones could result in a normal finding—a **false negative**, meaning there is something wrong, but it is mistaken as normal (figure 18).

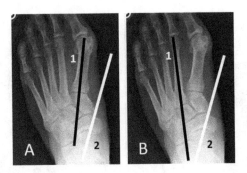

Figure 18. (A) Bisection of a misaligned first metatarsal bone (1) compared to the anklebone (2). This would be considered a normal measurement, even though the anklebone is partially dislocated. (B) Bisection of the second metatarsal bone (1) compared to the bisection of the anklebone (2). This shows a pathologic ankle.

Talar-Second Metatarsal Angle

The **talar-second metatarsal angle** is the angle between the anklebone and the second metatarsal. This is the most accurate angular measurement between the hindfoot and the forefoot. The second metatarsal bone serves as the reference point to the forefoot because it is more stable than the first metatarsal bone. There are varying degrees of acceptable measurement of the T2MA, but it is generally agreed that an angle less than 16 degrees is considered normal (figure 19, photo A) and that values greater than 16 should be considered abnormal (figure 19, photo B).[36]

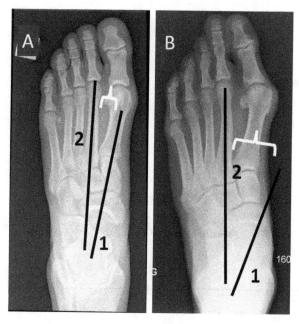

Figure 19. (A) Normally aligned hindfoot and forefoot. The bisection of the ankle (1) is compared to the bisection of the second metatarsal bone (2). (B) Partially displaced anklebone. Notice the increased angle between the bisection of both bones.

Ankle Bone-Navicular Alignment

The head of the anklebone should be firmly connected to the base of the navicular bone. If the anklebone turns inward and loses some of the joint contact, this also is an indication of abnormal anklebone alignment and of instability on the heel bone, which will lead to increased strain on the inner soft tissue of the arch.

Remember when we learned about the importance of the alignment of the first metatarsal bone? If the first metatarsal bone is angled away from the second metatarsal bone, the forefoot will turn outward, placing strain on the inner soft tissue when walking, standing, or running.

You have probably caught on by now that there are many different alignment issues with the bones that can lead to increased strain to the inner soft tissues. This is a recurring theme and very important in the diagnosis and treatment of chronic heel pain.

Alignment of the Big-Toe Joint

As with lateral-view X-rays, the last area to look at in the DP view is the big-toe joint. We want to see a nice, clear space between the head of the first metatarsal and the base of the big-toe bone (figure 20). If there is a larger-than-normal deviation between the first and second metatarsal bones, this could also lead to increased strain to the plantar fascia. If there is barely a space or lots of **fuzzy bone spurs**, this means there is arthritis of the big-toe joint, which will alter the way you walk. The big-toe joint needs to bend as you walk; if it can't, your body will compensate for limited motion of the big-toe joint by turning your forefoot outward. Guess what this can lead to? You're right: increased strain to the inner soft tissues on the bottom of your foot!

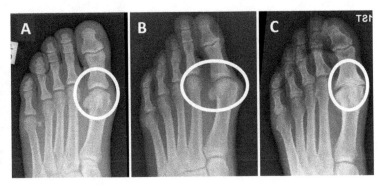

Figure 20. (A) Normal big-toe joint. (B) Misaligned big-toe joint. (C) Arthritic changes to the big-toe joint, with loss of normal range of motion.

Wow, you did it! Now that you've learned what to look for in a lateral-view X-ray of the foot, you are on your way to looking at an X-ray to see many things that most medical professionals may not take into consideration when diagnosing heel pain. Great job!

What I have presented here are just a few of the most important landmarks that a foot specialist will observe on your X-rays. It is important for them to factor any abnormal finding into your treatment planning. Because the foot is so complex, there could be many faulty parts that will need to be addressed in working toward the goal of restoring your foot structure to reduce the strain on the plantar fascia.

Ultrasonic Imaging

Some physicians will want to visually examine the soft tissues of your heel. This type of imaging isn't always considered essential in the *diagnosis* of heel pain, but it can help guide *treatment*. This is a cost-effective method (when compared to an **MRI**) to evaluate the thickness of the plantar fascia and to monitor the effect of treatment.[37]

It has been suggested that thickening of the plantar fascia by more than five millimeters should be considered pathologic.[38,39] But it has also been shown that people can have a thicker plantar fascia without any heel pain, and others have thinner plantar fascia with heel pain.[40,41] Zhang et al. studied young and elderly volunteers, and their findings showed increased thickness in the older subjects versus the younger ones.[42]

The thickness or thinness of the plantar fascia will not change the recommended form of treatment. There is nothing wrong with a physician wanting to document the thickness; it just doesn't help with determining the underlying cause to your heel pain: faulty foot mechanics.

Misaligned Feet and Chronic Heel Pain

To analyze the problem, we have begun by creating the "what's broken" list. Your doctor does this while taking your medical history and performing the physical and radiological exams of your foot. We have seen that many factors must be taken into consideration to finally come to a diagnosis for heel pain. What's really important to the medical specialist is discovering the underlying cause of your heel pain.

Once we have made sure there are no fractures, bone tumors, nerve entrapments, or other more uncommon issues, we must conclude that the faulty foot structure—specifically a misaligned anklebone and/or other bones and joints of your foot—has led to increased strain to the plantar fascia.[43–55]

Putting the Puzzle Together

We learned earlier that, essentially, the inner band of the plantar fascia connects the heel to the ball of the foot; that **inner column of the foot/** inner arch is unstable and has more motion than it should. The ankle-bone is responsible for locking and unlocking the bones of the foot, and when the anklebone loses its stability, that leads to a lowering of the inner arch. While standing, walking, or running, excessive strain is placed first on the innermost fibers of the plantar fascia.

This flexible hindfoot deformity begins occurring when the person starts walking. Multiply that by forty years of walking, and that results in greater than seventy million steps taken in the average lifestyle— and people who walk or run for exercise can dramatically increase that number. Finally, a critical threshold is reached, and the strong fibers just can't tolerate the forces anymore; the fibers snap, just like a broken rubber band.

The plantar fascia was able to withstand the strain for a while, but eventually, it could no longer withstand those excessive forces, and it developed **micro-ruptures**. (Think of this like overstretching a rubber band many times until it breaks.) At that point, the surrounding cells reacted by thickening and trying to repair and strengthen the weakened tissues. The thickened tissue pushing on the nerves is the key ingredient in the recipe for pain.

It's not your fault that you developed heel pain. What is at fault is loss of stability of those hindfoot bones. You have to also think about the cumulative effect of walking on a weakened foot structure day after day (figure 21). Did you know that the average person has taken more than seventy million steps by forty years of age (figure 22)? That's seventy million times the inner band to the plantar fascia has been overstretched. It's no wonder that the most common age to develop plantar fascia damage is forty.[56,57]

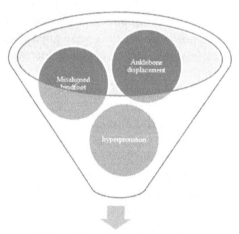

Excessive strain to the plantar fascia

Figure 21. "Recipe" for heel pain.

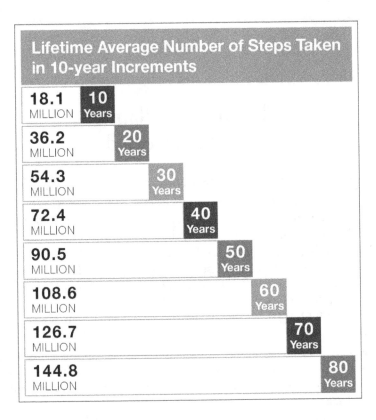

Figure 21. Number of steps taken per decade.

The Myth of Plantar Fasciitis Revealed

The use of the term "plantar fasciitis" is misleading and is the reason why heel pain has been one of the most challenging tissue disorders to treat. The attachment of **-itis** to the end of a word is an indication that an inflammatory condition is occurring, as with bursitis, arthritis, and gastroenteritis. In this case, it means that there is an inflammation of the plantar fascia: **fasciitis** (*fah-she-eye-tis*). This term is known and may forever be associated with heel pain, but medical research has proven that there is no inflammation.

NEWS FLASH: An inflammatory process does *not* actually occur within the plantar fascia, meaning this term, "plantar fasciitis," is not accurate for pain in the plantar fascia. You may ask why this is important because, if you have this condition, you probably don't care what it is called—you just want to get rid of your pain so you can get your life back.

The answer to this question is extremely important, however. If this plantar fasciitis is an inflammatory problem, then a simple regimen of anti-inflammatory treatments should easily resolve the condition. Many scientific studies of the fascia of patients with chronic heel pain have been undertaken. Amazingly, all of these studies independently revealed a lack of inflammation.[58–62] That tells us that there actually is no inflammation; there is a whole other disease process occurring instead. This could explain why it takes such a long time for most patients' heel pain to "go away": The prescribed treatments are used to address inflammation, rather than the real cause of the heel pain.

The **myth** is that chronic heel pain is due to an inflammation of the plantar fascia. There is *no* inflammation of the fascia, however. The surrounding tissues may become inflamed, but the fascia itself is not. Professional athletes have had their careers cut short because they were given treatments that were focused on an inflammation of the plantar fascia, and little was done to properly address their faulty foot structure. Think about the hundreds of millions of healthcare dollars that have been wasted on trying to "fix" an inflammation that wasn't even present.

If it's not inflammation, then what is it, Doc?

The real fascia problem is an -osis, not an -itis.

After the unusual, less common causes of heel pain have been ruled out, we can discover the real underlying reason why you've developed this heel pain. If it's not an inflammation, then what is it?

It's been known for quite a while that, as mentioned earlier, the real cause of this chronic heel pain condition is the repetitive micro-trauma overload injury, rather than an inflammation problem. The leading cause of chronic heel pain is years, even decades, of excessive strain on and overstretching of the plantar fascia due to a **misaligned hindfoot**.[63–77]

So, the fascia and other structures must somehow deal with those extra forces, or the fibers will start to rupture. The plantar fascia will try to heal itself, which it can do if given enough time and if the deforming forces have been minimized. But what if those deforming forces *aren't* minimized? Those excessive forces will take their toll.

Before we go any further, we must ask ourselves what would cause an **overloading** of the plantar fascia, because we must always eliminate, as much as possible, the source of the overstretching; otherwise, we may never permanently end this condition.

What Is the Role of a Flat or Misaligned Foot?

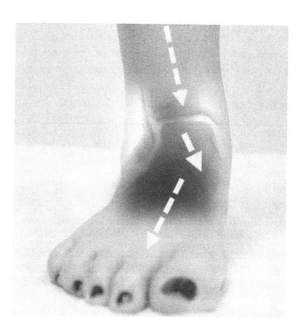

A flat or lower than normal arch does not guarantee you will develop chronic heel pain. However, most people with chronic heel pain have a lower than normal arch or a misaligned hindfoot, because there are only so many ways the structures of your foot can compensate for faulty foot mechanics. Eventually, something's got to give, and that's why flat feet lead to many problems in the body, including heel pain.

What is surprising to many **clinicians** is that many patients with heel pain have normal-appearing arches. **Plantar fasciosis**, the overstretching of the plantar fascia, can occur in both lower- and normal-appearing arches. The reason for this has to do with the angle of the heel bone and the stability of the navicular bone. The heel may have a normal or even higher than normal angle, which prevents a lowering of the arch, yet the anklebone sitting on top of the heel can still shift forward and inward, increasing the strain on the plantar fascia during walking. That explains why not all patients with chronic heel pain have flat feet.[78,79]

Foot Mechanics 101

Now you are going to learn about the phases of walking. Get ready to become a foot **biomechanics** specialist!

Walking is an amazing engineering miracle that we take for granted. It involves the coordination of many different parts of the body, and it all happens without us really thinking about it. We just get up and go. This section will tell you why the mechanics of your feet—especially the alignment and stability of your anklebone—are so important.

Gait cycle is the medical term for walking. There are two main phases of walking: **swing** and **stance**. In the swing phase, the foot is in the air, or is non-weightbearing, and in the **stance phase**, the foot is touching the ground or another weightbearing surface.

During the swing (noncontact) phase of the walking cycle, your foot is in the air, swinging forward until it touches the ground surface. While in the air, the anklebone is aligned with the heel and navicular bones, and the joints are aligned, putting no stress on the arch or the plantar fascia.

The stance phase, when the foot touches the ground, is divided into heel strike, stance (early/late), heel lift, and finally, toe-off (figure 23).

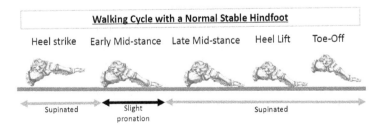

Figure 23. Walking cycle with a normal stable hindfoot.

The outer back of the heel or shoe is the first part that should come into contact with the ground surface. The ankle joints should be aligned on the heel bone and navicular bone, and the sinus tarsi should be in an open position.

As the walking cycle continues, the rest of the bottom of the foot will come into contact with the ground surface. During this time, the anklebone turns slightly inward, and the rest of the foot turns slightly outward. This is the pronation motion, which you'll remember is an important unlocking of the joints of the foot so they can quickly adapt to an uneven ground surface, if necessary. The maximum pronation, or weakening of the foot bones, occurs at approximately 38 percent of the foot contact with the ground, right at the end of early mid-stance.[80] At that point, the anklebone should switch direction and rotate outward (supination motion) to "relock" the joints of the foot. This changes the foot from a weak sack of bones to a strong, rigid structure. The weight of the body moves from the hindfoot (at heel strike) and passes through the forefoot, mid-stance, until the toes lift off the ground, toe-off, and are in the air again.

The orientation of the joint surfaces of the heel bone are guided by the ligaments between the anklebone and the leg bones (**tibia**, **fibula**), heel, and navicular bones.[81] There are no tendons attached to the anklebone. Excessive anklebone motion occurs because of an abnormality of the joint surfaces.

The plantar fascia is a major stabilizing structure of the inner arch of the foot during the weightbearing part of the walking cycle.[82] The maximum strain on the plantar fascia occurs during the latter part of the walking cycle, especially when the heel is lifted off the ground (figure 24).[83] Running creates increased stresses on the plantar fascia—a lot more than just with ordinary walking. That's why heel pain is a very common symptom in runners.[84] When you run, the forces acting on the plantar fascia are transferred to the forefoot, which compresses the joints of the inner arch.[85] There is a stretching strain on the plantar fascia during pronation of the foot, and a recoil of the foot that functions like a spring occurs during supination.[86] There is a release of "stored" energy in the foot as the heel is lifted and the ball of the foot is pushed off the ground.[87]

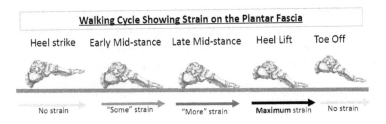

Figure 24. Walking cycle showing the amount of strain acting on the plantar fascia.

The hindfoot bones are vertical, and the forefoot bones are horizontal. This creates a slight twisting mechanism when walking. As the leg moves forward, the ankle joint bends, and the foot remains on the ground. This is like pulling the end of a spring. Bending the toes upward pulls the spring even more, and once the ball and toes of the foot leave the ground, the spring snaps back into its normal position, propelling the foot forward.[88] An increased, excessive, or prolonged period of pronation will lead to increased forces acting on the plantar fascia.

Alignment and Stability of the First Metatarsal Bone

Bending the big toe is the primary force that applies a strain to the inner band of the plantar fascia when the heel is lifted off the weight-bearing surface.[89,90] As you'll remember from previous chapters, other factors that can increase the strain on the inner band of the plantar fascia are the stability or instability and the alignment or misalignment of the first metatarsal bone. (Just in case you forgot from our previous discussion, that's the long bone behind the big toe.) When the heel leaves the ground, forces to the forefoot can exceed the body's weight by 20 percent.[91]

Anklebone instability = prolonged pronation = increased strain on the inner tissues of the plantar fascia.

If too much pronation occurs within the foot, this will lead to increased strain to the inner band of the plantar fascia (figure 25).[92,93] One of the reasons this increases strain has to do with the flexibility of the toe joints. Carlson et al. showed that increased motion of the toe joints increases the strain on the plantar fascia and increases the pull on the **Achilles tendon**.[94] Overpronation makes the forefoot turn outward, and this leads to an increase in the pressures on the toe joints and, therefore, increases the strain and mechanical overloading on the plantar fascia (figure 26).[95,96]

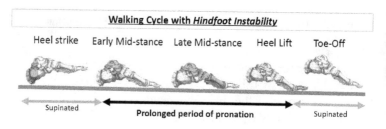

Figure 25. Walking cycle with partial dislocating anklebone.

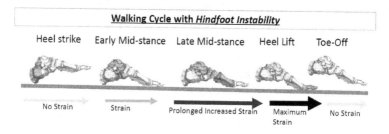

Figure 26. Walking cycle showing excessive amount of strain on the plantar fascia.

This chapter may have been a bit tough to follow, but the information is very important to understand when considering treatment options to decrease the excessive strain on the plantar fascia. I hope by now you truly understand how the instability of the anklebone increases the strain on the plantar fascia.

Plantar Fasciitis May Be a Myth, but My Heel Pain Is Real!

S kin, ligaments, blood vessels, tendons, and muscles all have nerve endings monitoring these tissues. There are nerve branches that pierce through the plantar fascia as they make their way to the skin receptors on the bottom of the foot. It is believed that the **micro-tears**, along with the thickening of the plantar fascia (fasciosis), lead to compression and damage to these **nerve fibers**.[97,98] Nerves don't like to be compressed or stretched, so they give you a signal that something is wrong. That signal is pain.

Rarely is the site of pain located exactly where the plantar fascia fibers insert into the heel bone. Rather, the center point of pain is from several millimeters to a centimeter beyond the insertion point of the fibers into the bottom of the heel bone. The plantar fascia, as we now know, has to counter, or resist, overstretching because when any tissue in the body is overstretched, it naturally wants to **contract** to prevent those forces. Talk to anyone who has undergone arthroscopic knee surgery; the knee joint has been pulled apart so the camera and other instruments can be inserted into the joint. After the procedure, patients complain of limited range of motion/bending of the knee joint. This is because the ligaments, tendons, and muscles contract because of the overstretching.

The only time the plantar fascia is *not* overloaded is when a person is sitting or lying down. When you stand, walk, or run during the day, overloading of the plantar fascia occurs, and it is overstretched (figure 27). The fascia tissue thickens as a reaction to the mechanical overloading. It is trying to get stronger to deal with the excessive pulling. There will be an increase in blood flow to the fascia.[99] When you get off your feet, the fascia, no longer weightbearing, naturally contracts, especially when you are sleeping and have been off your feet for several hours.

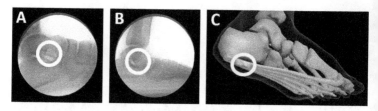

Figure 27. (A) the sinus tarsi is open, and the anklebone is aligned just prior to the heel touching the ground. As the entire bottom of the foot contacts the ground (B), the anklebone partially dislocates, closing the sinus tarsi. Immediately, an increased strain is placed on the plantar fascia with every step taken (C).

It takes longer than overnight, however, for the fascia to heal any micro-tears; when you get up during the night or in the morning, you have pain in your heel because the tissues are again overstrained. Throughout the day, the same forces as from the previous day continue to act on the heel, and so the cycle of the plantar fascia overstretching and contracting ensues—until there is a decrease of the mechanical overstretching long enough for the fascia to heal or until the band of fascia tissue ruptures completely.

Inferior Calcaneal Nerve Can Be a Real Pain!

A specific nerve—the inferior calcaneal nerve (ICN)—has been implicated as the culprit of heel pain.[100–103] Specifically, it is a branch from the main nerve traveling behind the inner anklebone and below the heel. It supplies sensory information from the heel bone, as well as helps to control some of the small muscles in the arch. It is this nerve that will signal the pain, but after a person has walked for a while, the compression force on the nerve shuts down the nerve impulses and creates a nerve disease called **neuropathy**.[104–106]

A study by Mizuno et al. found that the ICN is sometimes different in men and women.[107] Many MRI and **ultrasound** studies have shown thickening of the plantar fascia in the area of this nerve branch.[108,109] Those thick, tough fibers will compress the nerve, which, just like a person standing on a garden hose, will stop the nerve impulses from flowing, so the heel pain subsides.[110,111] But as time goes on, if the tissue doesn't heal, nerve damage will actually occur, until there is constant pain. This explains why "first-step pain" occurs: There was no pressure on the nerve, and then there *is* pressure.

Many treatments have involved nerve destruction or surgical **excision** of the nerves to the inner heel. These treatments will be discussed in a later chapter, but the important factor to our current discussion is the short-term improvement. A numbing medication (local anesthetic) injected into the inner heel provides pain relief because it disables the nerves from sensing pain. Because you've been really paying attention to this book, you will conclude that it is the numbing medication, *not* the **steroid** that gives pain relief.

As we already know from earlier chapters, it is extremely important to properly diagnose a problem, because a wrong diagnosis will lead to ineffective forms of treatment. It is surprising to me that many medical professionals know that an inflammatory process is not present with inner heel pain, yet still recommend treatments to address the inflammation while doing little to fix the underlying cause. In chapter 11, we're going to discuss the treatments that are recommended to treat heel pain, along with the research that shows less-than-desired results.

Doc, Be Honest: How Bad Is It?

As with any disease process, for heel pain, it is important to discover the extent and severity of damage in order to provide the best treatment. The sooner you seek medical treatment, the better/faster (hopefully) the condition will go away. The factors that predict how long it will take are discussed below:

A. **Whether this is the first or second (or later) episode of heel pain**

   The first episode should be easier to treat than the second time you develop heel pain. The second episode will take much longer to fix.

B. **If the heel pain occurs only in the morning, when you first get out of bed, and for how long**

   The time it takes for the heel pain to go away is a potential indicator of the degree of tissue damage.

C. **If the heel pain occurs two or more times a day after the foot has been non-weightbearing for more than thirty minutes**

   This is a more serious form of heel pain that is usually associated with the second episode of heel pain. It indicates more tissue destruction than if pain happens only once in the morning.

D. **If the heel pain occurs all the time, with every step taken**

   This is an indicator that there is significant nerve and tissue damage. This is an "end-stage" scenario, meaning that invasive measures are needed to fix the pain, and the chance of it going away on its own is extremely thin.

E. **How long you have had the pain**

   The longer the heel pain has been present, the longer it's going to take to go away.

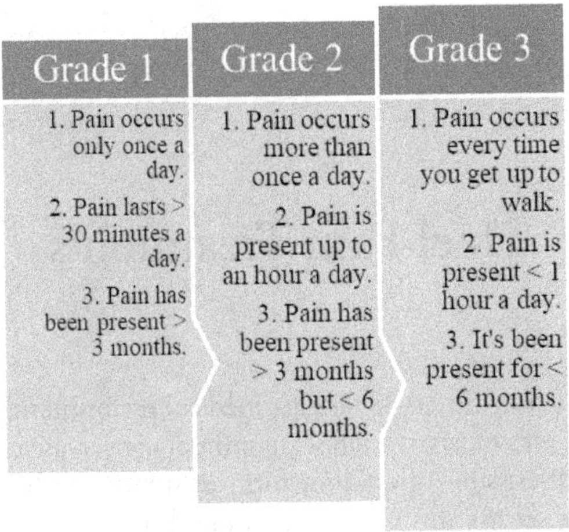

Grade 1	Grade 2	Grade 3
1. Pain occurs only once a day. 2. Pain lasts > 30 minutes a day. 3. Pain has been present > 3 months.	1. Pain occurs more than once a day. 2. Pain is present up to an hour a day. 3. Pain has been present > 3 months but < 6 months.	1. Pain occurs every time you get up to walk. 2. Pain is present < 1 hour a day. 3. It's been present for < 6 months.

Figure 28. Graphic showing three levels of heel pain.

The reason it's important to have a grading or classification system (figure 28) is to know how bad of a situation we're dealing with. If you experience more pain several times a day for several months, we're dealing with a more severe situation (i.e., Grade 3)—not life-threatening, of course, but most likely the foot will exhibit scar tissue, the nerves will be damaged, and it will take longer to heal.

12

Heel-Pain Treatments

F or a very long time—too long—medical recommendations were that patients must undergo six months of conservative care before there was discussion of another form of intervention (figure 29). That meant six months of limping around on a very painful heel, the patient's quality of life suffering, and "treatments" geared only to fixing an inflammation that wasn't even present. Let's look now at the most common forms of heel-pain treatments.

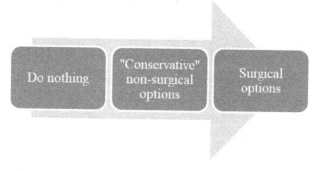

Figure 29. There are three main treatment options for heel pain.

As we've covered previously, if you are going to treat a condition, you need to know what you are trying to fix. Currently, the majority of treatments meant to "cure" heel pain are directed toward alleviating an inflammatory process. Patients are told to take anti-inflammatories, ice their heels, and stretch out their arches, and they are given heel injections. Sometimes, mild forms of this condition may respond to these forms of conservative therapy. There is a high likelihood, however, that the heel pain will come back—it's not *if*, it's *when*.

Observation: The Do-Nothing Approach

Many medical professionals feel that no treatment for heel pain is necessary.[112] One study has shown that a significant number of patients were "healed" with just conservative care.[113] We must take a closer look at that study, however. The mainstream medical community is happy to tell anyone with this condition that it will most likely take nearly a year—or even longer—for this condition to go away.[114] If you are a patient of one of these doctors and you have heel pain, you are reminded with every step that you have pain. This is going to severely affect your quality of life. You are going to decrease your activity level, which can lead to a decrease in metabolism and an increase in weight, and you will alter the way you walk, which can lead to overuse injuries to your knees, hips, or back.[115]

How does this condition just magically "heal" itself? It really depends on the severity of the micro-tears in the first place. Let's say you just started walking for exercise, and within a short period of time, you developed the heel pain. You stopped walking for exercise, eliminating the additional source of mechanical overload, and the fascia was able to heal itself. Your reward for trying to exercise was pain. Since the pain resolved and you were once more motivated to exercise, you began walking for exercise again. Because the underlying cause of the tissue strain—the faulty foot mechanics—is still present, however, it will only be a matter of time before the heel pain returns.

We've discussed previously that when you do have recurrence of heel pain, you are going to have a real challenge on your hands, because the fascia has many micro-tears and it is possible that there is scar tissue from the previous episode, making it less likely for the condition to resolve on its own this time. Many patients are told to just keep walking and one day the pain will go away. If you wait long enough, it probably *will*, but then your foot, leg, and back can also become affected.

By now, because you've stuck with me this long, you know that there are excessive forces acting on the inner arch of the foot, which leads to overstretching of the inner band of the plantar fascia. Micro-tears continue to develop, and excessive overloading continues with every step. The healing cells that are trying to repair those tears are busy at work, but they are fighting a losing battle. Damage to the tissue occurs when walking, and healing will occur only when there is no more strain to the tissue (i.e., when you're off your feet). The cells accumulate around the micro-tears like a callus on your skin to protect and strengthen the tissue. This thickness has a benefit, but it also will lead to compression of the nerves trapped between the plantar fascia and the heel bone. Those nerves will become damaged, and they will send a signal to the brain that something is wrong. That signal is pain in the heel.

If the healing cells are not able to compete with the strain on the tissue, then eventually, the plantar fascia will rupture and lose their ability to support the inner arch of the foot. There can be a few days of increased pain. Because the tissues have detached, however, there is no pressure on the nerves, so the nerves stop signaling pain, and you no longer have heel pain. That is the basis for physicians to say, "Wait it out," because eventually, the fibers could rupture on their own or the healing cells could bridge the gap between the micro-tears. But the end result is that the plantar fascia will now be elongated and the function to support the inner arch could be lost.

The big problem with elongated or partially ruptured fibers of the plantar fascia is that the foot has lost a major supporting structure of the inner arch. Imagine the supporting structure of a bridge being cut; the forces that were acting on that structure are now acting on other supporting structures, which are already handling mechanical overload. In the same way, the other structures within the foot may be able to handle these forces for some time, but there is a limit, and other aches and pains will eventually result.

Therefore, observation that offers no treatment amounts, essentially, to a medical professional standing on the sideline, watching and hoping. Heel pain is not a life-and-death situation, and it is okay to give your body a chance to heal without any medical intervention, but this chance for the body to heal itself should be short and only for a mild *first* case of heel pain.

Nonsurgical Treatments

It is often recommended that someone experiencing heel pain attempt three to six months of nonsurgical care prior to any surgical intervention. This seems to make sense, because who wants surgery if they don't need it, especially if the surgical procedure is somewhat radical (i.e., detaching the inner band of the plantar fascia and remolding the bottom of the heel bone)? There are potential risks and complications with every surgical procedure.

The important point to remember, though, is that conservative care does little to eliminate the excessive strain to the plantar fascia. Conservative care, for the most part, only attempts to ameliorate the symptoms. Here is a critical look at some very common conservative treatments.

Ice Therapy

The use of ice has been shown to have a benefit—in helping reduce inflammation. But remember from our earlier discussion that with chronic plantar fasciitis, we are not dealing with inflammation of the plantar fascia. Ice does provide other therapeutic advantages, such as decreasing nerve activity, but what does the ice do to prevent the excessive strain to the plantar fascia? Nothing. The application of ice is soothing but not **curative**. It's an afterthought. Imagine that you hit your thumb with a hammer. You apply ice, and that makes it feel better. What if you keep hitting your thumb with a hammer day after day? How is the ice helping? Shouldn't you just stop hitting your thumb with the hammer?

The main benefit of ice for your heel pain is that it compels you to be *off* your foot when you are applying the ice, essentially decreasing the strain to the plantar fascia with rest.

The real question, however, which this book repeatedly asks (and with good reason), is this: Can this treatment eliminate the excessive stress to the inner band of the plantar fascia? The answer, of course, is no. The goal needs to first be to decrease the strain to the plantar fascia, then to reduce symptoms.

Shoes and Shoe Gear

This isn't a book about shoes, but to not discuss shoes would be like writing a book about car problems and never discussing the tires. If you owned a luxury sports car, you probably would not put the cheapest tires you could find on it. Your feet are more valuable than a sports car, and I'd like you to make sure you're wearing good, supportive shoes. That doesn't mean women have to throw out those beautiful pumps, but if you're going to be doing a lot of walking, wear sensible shoes. You can always change shoes when you get to where you're going.

The types of shoes worn during your heel pain can help or hinder treatment. A study by Lin et al. showed that appropriate footwear can decrease the strain on the plantar fascia more than the type of arch support the patient wears.[116] People with heel pain should avoid flat or low-heel shoes because, as we discussed earlier, a shoe with little or no heel height increases the strain to the plantar fascia. A shoe with a one-inch heel decreases the strain acting on the fascia. Men, it can be difficult for you to find a one-inch heel, so I recommend that you buy a pair of cowboy boots.

If you don't believe that a flat shoe increases the strain on your foot, you can see for yourself when you walk barefoot or walk with flip-flop-style shoes. You will quickly learn that this increases the pain to your inner heel.

Ideally, anyone who has chronic heel pain should wear at least a good supportive sneaker beginning as soon as they get out of bed in the morning and continuing until they go to bed at night.

Do you inspect your shoes? Here is a homework assignment: Go to wherever you keep your shoes and inspect them. You could have the best forms of treatment, but if you go back to wearing the same old, worn-out shoes … well, do you think that the treatment is going to be as effective as it was intended to be? Probably not!

In addition to the *type* of shoe, the *quality* of the shoe is important. The quality of materials used to make shoes isn't as high as it used to be, and shoes don't last as long as they used to. The outer heel wears out first. Please check the outer corners of the heels of the shoes you wear most. Find those shoes and put them on the counter (please place them on a piece of paper so you don't get any debris on your counter). You will see that it looks like someone took a file to the outer corner of each heel. When you wear these worn-out shoes, it increases the strain on the plantar fascia.

Shoes just aren't made as well as they were years ago. While the top and sides of the shoe might look and feel great, the outer bottom part of the heel gets worn out. Imagine having four to seven times your body weight landing on the back of your heel thousands of times per day. Eventually, the heel wears out. This forces your heel to turn outward, placing increased stress on the inner-arch tissues of the foot.

Do your feet (and possibly your knees, hips, and back) a favor, and either repair or throw away worn-out shoes!

If you have a mild case of heel pain and it's a first-time occurrence, it is possible that just by wearing a new pair of shoes, you will eliminate the excessive strain—and voila! Your heel pain will shortly disappear. Unfortunately, if it's your second time around and your pain lasts for more than one hour a day, you are going to need more than a new pair of shoes to get rid of your heel pain.

The theory of having patients with heel pain wear shoes with one- or two-inch heels is to try to take strain off the plantar fascia by raising the heel. This method is controversial, however. Yu et al. found a positive effect from decreasing plantar fascia strain, but also an increased risk of ankle ligament injury.[117] Another study found that the plantar fascia strain did not increase with low heels and concluded that the influence of heel elevation itself did not make a difference, but it was the stability of the inner arch structure that decreased the strain to the plantar fascia.[118] The authors of these studies cautioned against recommending heel elevation in the treatment of heel pain, because an elevated heel would not decrease the strain on the plantar fascia.

One of the implicating factors for the development of heel pain is a tight Achilles tendon or calf muscle.[119–121] The fascia tissue does have a connection with the lining (**paratenon**) of the Achilles but has no connection to the Achilles tendon itself.[122] The connection is mainly with the lining of the heel bone (periosteum).

Wearing a shoe with more than a one-inch heel height could also help to compensate for a tight Achilles tendon or calf muscle, but this still does not address the anklebone misalignment and instability. It is possible that an increased heel height will decrease the strain on the fascia enough so the fascia can heal, but the underlying problem still exists, and there is an increased risk that the heel pain will reoccur.

Oral Medication(s)

We live in a society that has been brainwashed to believe that pills are the answer to any medical condition. A cross-sectional study using the National Ambulatory Medical Care Survey data from 2000 to 2007 found that the annual cost of medications prescribed to adults for pain was $17.8 billion dollars.[123] Every single pill has potential side effects, and the longer you take the pill, the more likely you will develop a side effect. The problem is that we as patients have become too accustomed to just taking that pill as the extent of our participation. The truth is that the more you are involved in your medical care, the more successful the outcome will be.

Pills by themselves certainly cannot solve the mechanical overloading of the plantar fascia, and several studies have shown that there is no significant benefit—and even potential risks—with this form of treatment.[124] We know that there isn't a genuine inflammatory condition of the fascia, so an anti-inflammatory pill won't help fix the underlying problem. A pain pill will temporarily knock out or decrease the signal that the pain sensor sends out. There is pain, however; something somewhere is stimulating a pain sensor to signal pain.

Injections

Thousands of people every day receive injections into their painful heels. These injections typically contain an anesthetic mixed with a steroid. The anesthetic temporarily knocks out the involved nerves, stopping the pain, and the steroid helps to reduce tissue inflammation. Usually, local anesthesia can last an hour or even several hours after it has been given. Some patients may even get *days* of relief. Those who have greater tissue disease, however, may receive little to no relief.

What's so bad about receiving an injection for and experiencing relief from heel pain? I am glad you asked! Remember, the leading cause of plantar-fascia tissue damage is the mechanical overloading of the **central band of the plantar fascia**. A heel injection clearly does not eliminate the overloading of the fascia. Once the body's warning signal and protective mechanism—heel pain—has been temporarily knocked out, the person who received the injection may be elated. There have been many things they wanted to do but couldn't because of the pain, so now they go on a rampage—walking, shopping, doing yard work … you name it.

After a day or maybe several days, the injection finally wears off, and the heel pain is even worse than before. The person goes back to their doctor and states, "Well, it worked for a few days, but the pain came back." The doctor gives another injection, with the same results. Unfortunately, there is a limit to how many injections may be given. Most foot specialists will give up to only three injections— maximum—spread out over several months. In fact, it has been found that multiple injections of steroids into the heel can lead to the rupture of this fascia.[125–127]

Recent studies have been published comparing the injection of special anti-inflammatory medications to the typical **corticosteroid**.[128,129] These studies found no difference between the types of anti-inflammatory medicine. This further supports the fact that there isn't an inflammation to treat. An analysis of the effectiveness of the interventions in the management of chronic heel pain concluded that "steroid injection or iontophoresis may be useful, but of transient effect," which means it doesn't last long.[130] Another study, by Li et al., compared steroid injections to a placebo.[131] The authors warned that "corticosteroid injection may provide pain relief for a short period of time, but the efficacy may disappear with the progression of time." That's because the underlying etiology is still present.

Remember that the goal of treatment is to reduce or eliminate the excessive forces acting on the plantar fascia. How can this be accomplished with an injection of anesthesia or steroid? *It can't.*

A very extensive review of 765 patients with chronic plantar fasciosis showed that more than 51 percent developed a plantar fascia rupture as a result of combination of local anesthetic and steroid injections to treat their pain.[132] Such ruptures will lead to other long-term complications.

Injection of platelet-rich plasma (PRP) has become very popular in recent years as an optional form of treatment.[133] The idea is that within this solution drawn from the patient's blood are "healing cells." Although this injection technique has been useful for some forms of disease, a recent study has shown that it has the same effect as other injections on the plantar fascia.[134] One interesting study showed that patients who had an injection of the PRP had better foot function after the injection.[135] The study did not measure pain, however, only that patients were more active after the injection. It also didn't say just how active patients were or how long it took for them to improve. The study shows that there is at least some benefit in the short-term, but it was not a long-term study. The bottom line is that the mechanical overloading of the plantar fascia is still present even after a PRP injection. In addition, this kind of injection is also very costly and isn't always covered by insurance carriers.

Injection of **silicone** into the heel pad has been recommended by one group of doctors.[136] This study shows that people will try nearly anything to get rid of their heel pain. Of course, this treatment does not address the underlying etiology of excessive strain on the plantar fascia due to anklebone instability. Additionally, this treatment is not an option in the United States, at least at the time of this book's publication.

Taping/Strapping

Strapping, also known as low-Dye taping, involves the application of an adhesive tape to the bottom and sides of the affected foot. The goal is to decrease the flexibility of the arch and, thus, decrease the strain on the plantar fascia. In the short term, this has proven to be an effective treatment,[137,138] reducing both pronation and supination of the hindfoot.[139]

Unfortunately, many people have developed adhesive allergies and ended up with a skin rash after this type of treatment. This tape can and should be left on the foot for only a few days. In addition, it's difficult to tape your foot yourself or to have a nonqualified, untrained person reapply it, so a few other types of wraps have been developed. Some of them can be helpful, but none of them are as effective as tape applied by a specialist.[140]

Even though taping is helpful to decrease the strain on the fascia, it cannot help to realign and stabilize the anklebone[141] and cannot help to restore the arch of the foot.[142] This means that taping is only a temporary and, therefore, less-than-effective measure for fixing heel pain.[143,144]

Interesting to note, however, is that the application of low-Dye taping has been found to be superior to use of an arch support in changing the dynamics on the bottom of the foot.[145] Franettovich et al. found that the combination of an ankle brace and low-Dye taping was able to help support the soft-tissue structures on the inner arch, compared to no support (that is, a bare foot).[146] Some support is clearly better than no support, but to reiterate: Low-Dye taping still does not internally realign and stabilize the anklebone. As soon as the tape and brace are removed, the excessive forces are again acting on the plantar fascia. Nothing has been fixed; the underlying cause is still present.

Arch Supports and Foot Orthoses

Another very commonly prescribed remedy for heel pain is an arch support. This seems to make perfect sense: If you can prevent the arch from collapsing, there should be a decrease in strain to the central band of the plantar fascia. Many people claim relief with the use of arch supports; however, even more don't. If we take a critical look at how the arch support functions, we quickly learn why it simply is ineffective for most people, at least in the long term.

First, we have learned that the true reason for the development of pain is the mechanical overstretching of the plantar fascia, which occurs as a direct result of the partial **displacement** of the ankle and heel bones. We have to ask the question, how can something placed *below* the heel stabilize the anklebone *above* it? Is there any evidence that an arch support can realign, stabilize, and prevent the partial dislocation of the ankle and heel bones? The answer is no, an arch support cannot perform that function.[147]

Arch supports also have many other limitations, whether the supports are custom-made or not. One is the difficulty of finding a shoe that fits the device without pushing against the painful area and making heel pain worse. Another limitation of arch supports is that you must make sure you are wearing your shoes with the inserts. When you are not wearing your shoes or are wearing your shoes without the inserts, nothing is helping to decrease the excessive forces when walking.

A study by Kogler et al. found that supporting the inner arch of the foot actually increased strain on the plantar fascia.[148] This goes against the theory of using an arch support to help the plantar fascia. Another study compared various shoe inserts and found that there was little difference among them in decreasing the strain on the plantar fascia.[149] Although the main goal of an arch support is to decrease the strain to the plantar fascia, not a single study to date has shown that arch supports decrease the strain on the plantar fascia. In fact, one study by Fleischer et al. showed that patients did not have an improvement in their heel pain after using their "foot supports" for three months.[150]

A **meta-analysis** was completed a few years ago to study the different forms of realigning the foot using motion-control footwear, arch supports, and low-Dye taping.[151] The researchers found that low-Dye adhesive taping was more effective than custom-made arch supports or motion-control footwear. Although another study the same year showed that some patients got better after wearing their arch supports,[152] there is much variability from one arch support to another, and two limitations of this study were that it was short-term and that patients only *felt better*—they didn't have complete resolution of their pain. In other words, none of the patients were cured.

Yes, it may be feasible, depending on the amount and duration of damage to the plantar fascia, for an arch support to help a patient. In fact, if I were experiencing heel pain, I would attempt an arch support prior to having my plantar fascia cut (more on that option later).

Another study, this one by Yucel et al., recommended the use of a full-length insole as the first line of treatment, having found little difference between the results of steroid injections and the use of insoles.[153] Obviously, putting an insole in your shoe hurts less than an injection in a painful area of your heel, but it still doesn't remove the cause of the heel pain (figure 30). Even more importantly, Lin et al. concluded that the type of shoe worn has a greater effect on reducing the strain to the plantar fascia than does the type of insole worn.[154]

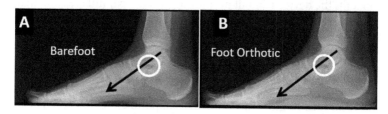

Figure 30. (A) Weightbearing X-ray of the foot showing anklebone displacement. (B) X-ray of the same foot, with a custom-made foot orthotic placed underneath. The anklebone is still displaced (misaligned).

Acupuncture

There is such a long list of "treatments" for heel pain because most treatments address the symptom—the pain—and when one doesn't work, people will try another, moving from one to the next, until they've tried just about everything. A study in 2011 comparing nonsurgical forms of heel-pain treatment found that some patients had some benefit with **acupuncture**.[155] The most important part to remember about this paper, however, was that acupuncture was never used as the *only* form of treatment; it was combined with many other forms of treatment. There have been positive benefits with the use of acupuncture in decreasing heel pain. Of course, we know that acupuncture cannot realign and stabilize the anklebone, and it cannot decrease the strain to the plantar fascia.

Stretching and Night-Resting Splints

Foot stretching has been a very popular conservative, nonsurgical recommendation. A study in 2003 showed that patients did better by performing non-weightbearing stretching of the plantar fascia than by stretching out their Achilles tendons.[156] A more recent study agreed with those findings: Wrobel et al. concluded that home Achilles tendon stretching may not be the best form of treatment, because patients with less severe tight Achilles tendons and less severe pain did worse with this form of treatment than did those with more severe pain.[157]

Another study concluded that a two-week stretching program "provides no statistically significant benefit in the 'first-step' pain, foot pain, foot function or general foot health compared to not stretching."[158]

An additional and rather common tool used in treatment of heel pain is the night splint. Barry et al. compared the use of night splints to the stretching of calf muscles and found that night splints functioned better than calf muscle stretches.[159] Splints are still not very helpful, however. The theory with these devices is that because the plantar fascia contracts when no weight is being placed on the foot, splints prevent this contracture and, therefore, help to eliminate the pain upon standing. Although this may be true for some patients, the majority of patients still experience overstretching of the plantar fascia while standing, so the working of the device is counterintuitive.

A good comparison that may help us understand is someone who keeps tapping their finger all day long. The finger hurts after the repetitive trauma that has been inflicted all day long, so at night the person places a brace on the finger, but again the next day, the same tapping occurs, so no real benefit is gained from the use of the brace.

Most patients find splints cumbersome to wear and impossible to sleep in, and even after using them religiously, patients see little to no benefit, so the splints eventually end up in the back of the closet. Splints are thus considered a short-term, temporary treatment that does nothing to decrease the strain on the plantar fascia or realign the anklebone.

Extended-Use Pulsed Radiofrequency Electromagnetic Field

For this treatment, a contraption worn on the heel intermittently sends sound-wave pulses into the tissues. Although one study showed that the treatment was helpful, it was not a long-term study.[160] Of course, this method is focused only on symptom relief, rather than on realigning and stabilizing the anklebone. (Remember, if we fix the cause, the symptom will go away!)

Extracorporeal Shockwave Therapy

There was once a lot of commotion about using shockwaves—the same kind of technology used to blast kidney stones—to break up the inflammation in the plantar fascia. Many papers were published about this mode of treatment.[161-164] Unfortunately, the mid- to long-term treatment didn't make much of an impact.[165]

One comparative study between shockwave therapy and heel surgery led the authors to recommend shockwave as a "reasonable earlier line of treatment of chronic plantar fasciitis" before heel surgery.[166] That was mainly because patients were able to walk immediately after shockwave therapy, without the complications of heel surgery, and were therefore able to resume activities sooner. The only problem with this study was the limited follow-up with the patients after the shockwave treatment: It was just a little over six months. The issue with shockwave therapy is—yes, you guessed it, and you are probably tired of hearing this—this treatment does not address the anklebone instability. Because the anklebone instability is not corrected, a patient's pain may improve initially, but because the underlying cause is not addressed, the excessive forces are still acting on the plantar fascia, and it's just a matter of time until the heel pain returns.

Low-Level Lasers

Some medical specialists have tried using **low-level laser** therapy to treat heel pain.[167] This sounds like an interesting and very modern technology. The questions remain, however: What does this treatment do to realign and/or stabilize the anklebone, and can it reduce the strain on the plantar fascia? Nothing, and of course not! That's why not all of the patients got better, even in the short term.

Immobilization

Many patients have been immobilized to correct their heel pain. With **immobilization**, a removable brace or even a lower-leg cast is applied to completely eliminate any motion of the foot and ankle. This can be an effective form of treatment at times, though it is very difficult for most patients to wear casts or braces on their legs for weeks at a time, for several reasons. They are not allowed to drive cars while wearing leg casts, they should not take showers while wearing leg casts, and it is very difficult to walk with a leg cast. Do I need to continue?

The reason this is an effective form of treatment is that it eliminates the mechanical overloading of the plantar fascia, giving the fascia a chance to heal because the nerves are no longer adversely affected. It can take several weeks to months, or even longer, for the fascia to heal, depending on the severity of involvement and all of the other factors associated with the grading/staging of this condition.

Although this form of treatment may provide resolution to the heel pain, I predict that it is only a temporary measure. Why? Again, what is the underlying cause of **plantar fasciopathy** in the first place? Mechanical overload of the plantar fascia. How does the application of a cast eliminate that mechanical overstretching of the plantar fascia once the cast has been removed? Was the patient's heel pain caused by wearing an old, worn-out pair of shoes and then running the Boston Marathon, or was it caused by years of a congenital hindfoot misalignment deformity?

Magnets

The use of magnets for pain relief has always been intriguing to me. This is a rather inexpensive treatment that is easy to use and has minimal side effects and no surgical or medication complications. It seems pretty straightforward. The only problem is that there just isn't any science to back it up.[168,169] I therefore do not recommend spending your hard-earned money on this form of "treatment."

Surgical Treatments for Chronic Heel Pain

There have been just as many surgical as nonsurgical treatments for heel pain. These range from minimally invasive to aggressive techniques, and research shows that the success rate of surgical intervention for chronic plantar fasciosis is low and that such intervention is associated with high complication rates and long recovery times.[170,171] Let's take a look at some of the most commonly recommended surgical treatments for chronic heel pain related to a diseased plantar fascia.

Radio-Frequency Nerve Ablation

Radio-frequency nerve ablation involves the insertion of an electrical probe into the deep tissues. An electrical impulse "zaps" the tissue, which shuts down and "reboots" any nerves in the area. A few studies have been published on this technique,[172–178] but there are no long-term follow-up studies. This technique does not realign and stabilize the anklebone, nor does it reduce the strain on the plantar fascia. Basically, it simply eliminates the associated pain. Meanwhile, the excessive abnormal forces continue to act on the foot.

Cryosurgery

Cryosurgery involves freezing the affected nerves.[179] It makes sense for pain management: Kill the nerves, and the pain will disappear. The only issue is that killing the nerves only addresses the symptoms, not the underlying etiology. This technique has pretty much fallen out of favor in recent years, which is just as well; with cryosurgery, as with nerve ablation, anklebone displacement is still present and will lead to other symptoms throughout the body. In a study by Cavazos et al. that followed 137 subjects for two years after surgery, thirty-one subjects had no improvement in their heel pain.[180] As you already know, it's better to fix the underlying cause than to simply freeze, kill, or cut out the nerves so patients don't notice the pain.

Plantar Fascia Release (Plantar Fasciotomy)

There are estimates that nearly one million people have had their plantar fascia cut (known as **plantar fasciotomy** or **plantar fascia release**), with or without a heel spur removed. One of my favorite sayings is

"Every solution has the potential to create a new problem." About the worst thing that someone can have done to their foot is the cutting of the most important structure supporting the arch of the foot. Instantly, the loss of support from the plantar fascia leads to increased strain to the **posterior tibial tendon**.[181–183] Eventually, this tendon becomes over-stretched and becomes ineffective to stabilize the inner arch bones. This tendon destruction causes **adult-acquired flat foot**.

Multiple studies have examined the outcome of plantar fasciotomy.[184–189] Surprisingly (or maybe not, if you've been paying attention so far), not all patients are cured of their pain after the plantar fascia has been cut; many patients who undergo this release continue to have heel pain. In many of those cases, it is possible that the pain only shifted to another part of the heel as a result.[190] Of course, because you have been reading this book, you immediately understand that the anklebone will still continue to partially dislocate and there will still be excessive forces acting on the inner column of the foot, both while standing and during every step taken.

In one study, Cheung et al. warned that only a minimal amount of the inner band of the plantar fascia be released, because there will be a much greater risk of the arch collapsing if more than that is cut.[191] They also showed that cutting the plantar fascia increases the strain to the other supporting structures of the foot. Forces shift to the outer part of the foot, arch height decreases, and there is increased strain to outer foot bones, specifically the cuboid (the bone in front of the heel bone).[6] Many other studies have also shown the negative effects of cutting the plantar fascia.[7] Many patients develop pain to the outer part of the foot after heel surgery. This pain is referred to as "cuboid syndrome" and is due to the increased strain to the outer midfoot from the loss of the stabilization effect of the plantar fascia.

Cutting of the plantar fascia can have a rather lengthy recovery and is associated with other complications, including persistent or recurrent acute heel pain, arch instability, and structural failure of the inner arch due to loss of stability.[192] Another lesser-reported complication of cutting the plantar fascia is the subsequent development of hammertoes.[193] One patient was even reported to have a fractured/broken metatarsal bone after the cutting of their plantar fascia.[194]

Yu et al. studied patients who had persistent pain after having the plantar fascia cut.[195] The researchers concluded that the continued pain was due to "recurrence of the plantar fasciitis, pathology related to arch instability, and structural failure from overload."

Sharkey et al. also conducted a study showing that **auto-rupture** or **surgical rupture** of the plantar fascia significantly increases the pressure under the second metatarsal head and can lead to a stress fracture.[196] They also showed that the forces to the ball of the foot are altered after rupture of the plantar fascia and that this could lead to **metatarsalgia**, or pain in the ball of the foot.

Yet another study also evaluated the surgical release of the plantar fascia and found a negative effect on the bones and arch of the foot after the release.[197] The researchers stated that there was also a negative effect on the heel bone and on the joint between the heel and cuboid.

So, does this procedure genuinely make any sense? What if you had chronic pain in the most powerful tendon in your body, the Achilles tendon? After a few months of nonsurgical treatment, would you allow your surgeon to simply cut and disconnect this tendon? I think the answer is no. But if you had chronic pain to your inner heel and your doctor told you, "Let's just cut the plantar fascia, and hopefully, the pain will go away," without truly knowing the potential negative outcome ... Well, you probably wouldn't be so quick to answer no.

We can see from all of these studies that many patients develop pain to the outer foot after the plantar fascia ruptures or is cut. The bottom line is that cutting the plantar fascia still does not address the underlying etiology of excessive motion in the anklebone.

Heel-Spur Removal

Heel pain has been blamed on a painful-looking bone formation on the bottom of the heel (calcaneus) called a heel spur. It is not normal to have a bony projection extending from the bottom tip of the heel. There is a tissue membrane on the covering of all bones called the **periosteum**. A weightbearing compressive force, with secondary tensioning of where the plantar fascia attaches to the heel, is the underlying cause of spur growth.[198,199] The bone "grows" in the direction of the tissue, pulling to shorten or ease the strain on the plantar fascia (figure 31).[200]

Probably because it is an abnormal finding, the heel spur was once thought, and unfortunately is still thought by many, to be the source of heel pain. This pointy prominence seen on an X-ray looks painful, but that is just supposition. The heel spur is falsely accused, and patients are told they will need surgery to remove it. You may be surprised to find out that many patients with heel pain don't have heel spurs visible on their X-rays. In fact, many people with heel spurs have never experienced heel pain.[201,202]

Researchers have actually discovered that patients with larger heel spurs respond to heel-pain treatment better than patients with smaller or nonexistent spurs.[203] This shows that the spur actually is a "good" finding because the spur is an attempt by the body to decrease the strain on the fascia.

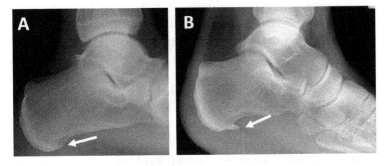

Figure 31. (A) Normal contour in the heel bone. (B) A heel spur.

So, if your X-ray reveals a heel spur, remember that **bone spurs** are found all over the body, and they are not always associated with pain. A heel spur is just a radiographic finding that, although looking like an impressive cause of heel pain, really *doesn't* cause heel pain or affect what treatment you need to fix your heel pain.

It used to be that the foot surgeon would want to immediately go in and remove heel spur(s) when a patient complained of chronic heel pain. Heel-spur removal, however, can decrease the success rate of eliminating heel pain.[204] In fact, there have been times when the removal of the heel spur has resulted in fracture of the heel bone.[205]

Although the spur extending from the heel bone *looks* painful on an X-ray, you don't actually walk *on* the spur itself, as it doesn't poke through the bottom of your heel; these sharp-looking spurs typically point forward, rather than down, and the heel spur actually develops because of degenerative changes that occur where the fascia attaches to the heel.[206]

A study by Osborne et al. compared X-rays of individuals with and without plantar fasciitis and found that 46 percent of patients who had never experienced heel pain had a heel spur and 85 percent of patients with heel pain did have a slight heel spur.[207] They concluded that the key radiological features that differentiated the group with heel pain were not the spurs but rather the changes in the soft tissues.

Besides the potential for fracture, there are other concerns with removing the bone spur. The only way to remove the spur is to completely detach the plantar fascia from the spur. The arch of the foot is weakened as a result, and the mechanical overloading of the foot is still quite present. Eventually, other supporting structures take up the tension and become symptomatic until they, too, need some form of reconstruction. In addition, the cutting of the fascia combined with removal of the bone spur leads to bleeding in that area that turns into a clot and can lead to more scar tissue thickening and fibrosis at the bottom of the heel bone, which could possibly lead to nerve **impingement** in that area.

Another study, by Jarde et al., showed an improvement of pain of only 75 percent in the short term for patients whose heel spurs were removed and that the patients noticed an increased sagging or lowering of their arches after the surgery.[208] Thus, after all the potential risks and complications of heel-spur removal, not all patients have resolution of their heel pain.

Surgical Lengthening of the Achilles Tendon

Many foot specialists feel that a tight Achilles tendon is the leading cause of chronic heel pain. They recommend cutting the tendon or some of the fibers that attach the tendon to the inner calf muscle, to allow the tendon to lengthen. Detaching the inner muscle attachment to the Achilles tendon decreases the strain on the Achilles tendon.

A study by Monteagudo et al. that compared cutting the plantar fascia with partial detachment of the Achilles tendon fibers to the inner calf muscle concluded that patients who had the Achilles tendon fibers released to the inner calf muscle had a faster recovery than those who had the plantar fascia cut.[209] Unfortunately, this was not a long-term study, so there's no way to determine how many patients' heel pain recurred or if those patients developed pain in other parts of their foot as a result of weakening the Achilles tendon.

What also needs to be understood here is this: A "lengthening," quite honestly, is achieved by cutting the tendon at certain angles that will allow its cut ends to gap open, creating tissue gap, or void. This weakens the tendon at the same time that it lengthens, and care must be taken so that the Achilles tendon does not completely rupture.

As one can certainly imagine, the cutting of the Achilles tendon is no picnic to heal from. Further, this approach doesn't always work, and it certainly does not address the true cause of the heel pain, which, as you now know, is faulty ankle and heel bone alignment.

Cutting and Shifting of the Heel Bone

A surgical procedure that is even more aggressive than lengthening of the Achilles tendon has been suggested as a form of treatment for chronic heel pain. This involves cutting the back end of the heel bone between where the Achilles tendon inserts and where the anklebone connects to the heel bone. In this procedure, surgeons shift the back end of the heel downward and inward in an attempt to help restore stability to the inner arch.

A study by Mivamoto et al. showed that many of the patients reported improvement in pain after the procedure.[210] It is possible that the strain to the plantar fascia stopped and the fascia was able to heal because of the prolonged time they had to stay off of their foot to recover from the surgery. No follow-up was done, however, to discover how long the patients remained pain-free. Furthermore, this procedure has not been shown to decrease the strain on the plantar fascia and has not been proven to realign and stabilize the anklebone.

Another study evaluated the cutting and shifting of the heel and also the insertion of a bone graft to the outer part of the heel bone.[211] They found that cutting and shifting the back of the heel made less of a change to the plantar fascia than did the insertion of the bone graft to the front of the heel.

Unfortunately, none of the treatments discussed in this chapter address the underlying etiology of chronic heel pain: **the instability and misalignment of the anklebone** (figure 32). These approaches to resolving heel pain account for the poor results experienced by the patients who undergo the procedures. In other words, as you now know from reading this book, more is at work in these patients' heel pain than is often assumed, and the opportunity to address the main cause of the pain is often missed. Heel pain can be truly resolved once the underlying *cause* is addressed—with EOTTS.

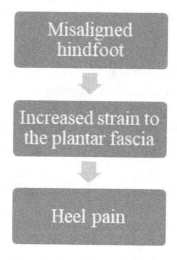

Figure 32. The etiology of heel pain.

EOTTS: The Missing Piece to the Plantar Fasciosis Treatment Puzzle

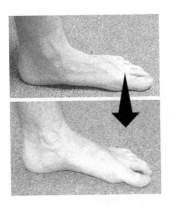
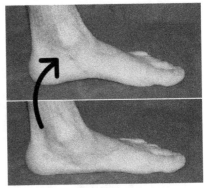

It is time to change our thinking. It is time to look at this medical issue in a whole new way—the right way and, certainly, the sensible way. Reject the myth of plantar fasciitis. It is time to simplify what has for far too long been a potentially arduous, unsuccessful, and exhausting process. It is time to treat this condition properly. It is time to finally attain the glory and gratification inherent in treating this problem accurately and with a success rate that we've clearly been seeking for too long:

extra-osseous talotarsal stabilization (EOTTS), a minimally invasive anklebone stabilization.

EOTTS is a superior option not discussed often enough. In fact, it is currently the best-kept secret in all of foot-and-ankle orthopedics. This is a minimally invasive outpatient (or even in-office) procedure in which a small titanium stent is inserted into the naturally occurring space between the ankle and heel bones (figure 32). (Remember the sinus tarsi discussed earlier?) It is similar to placing a stent into an artery to keep blood flowing.

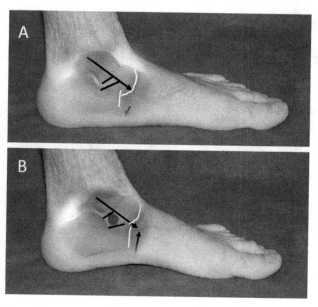

Figure 33. A photograph of a foot, with X-ray overlap, showing (A) anklebone displacement and (B) the improved angles and arch height after the insertion of a sinus tarsi implant.

This titanium stent, HyProCure, is the only device that has been scientifically proven to *immediately decrease the strain on the plantar fascia by 33 percent*.[212] Yes, this approach genuinely offsets the cause of chronic heel pain and works the best. No other form of treatment has been proven to decrease the strain acting on the innermost band of the plantar fascia.

As previously discussed, a congenital deformity can lead to the anklebone partially dislocating on the heel bone. When this happens, the anklebone turns inward and can slip forward, and the forces that should pass through the back of the heel instead act on the inner column of the foot bones. *This is the exact cause of the mechanical overloading of the central band of the plantar fascia.* There would be complete elimination of the strain to the fascia if the anklebone could be fused to the heel. Such fusing would be too drastic, though, as some motion needs to occur between these joints.

Titanium stents have been inserted with great success into the sinus tarsi of patients with chronic plantar fasciopathy. A long history of use of sinus tarsi implants demonstrates their safety and efficacy in both children and adults, and many scientific studies have shown positive outcomes.[213–228]

The benefits of this procedure clearly overshadow all of the symptom-based treatments discussed in this book. EOTTS simply makes sense. Because this is an *internal*, rather than *external*, option, the **sinus tarsi stent** works at all times, with or without shoes. There are no allergic reactions to the titanium, like there can be to adhesive tape. The stent is professionally inserted once and does not have to be repeatedly reapplied. Further, the sinus tarsi stents are proven to normalize abnormal radiographic angles, reset navicular bone position, and decrease forces acting on the inner column of the foot.

There are basically two types of sinus tarsi implants available. The type I **arthroereisis** (*are-throw-ear-ee-sis*) devices are placed into the outer portion of the sinus tarsi. Unfortunately, they have very high removal rates because the anklebone hits against them during walking and running. Eventually—usually by two to three years after they have been inserted—40 percent or more of patients with this type of implant will develop pain from the implant, requiring it to be removed. The type II **non-arthroereisis** device (HyProCure, GraMedica Macomb, Michigan) has been proven to be the best device, with long-term success rates of 94 percent. This device is placed more deeply and more centrally than the arthroereisis devices and, thus, prevents the anklebone from shifting from its desired position, while still allowing the normal range of motion.

The sooner the EOTTS procedure can be performed, the better, because it stops the problem at its root (figure 33). The EOTTS-HyProCure option addresses the underlying cause of heel pain, making it possible for other forms of conservative care to be able to work their "magic" on the symptoms. The longer one waits to have the EOTTS procedure, the more damage will occur to the plantar fascia, and the greater likelihood that the nerves will become permanently damaged.

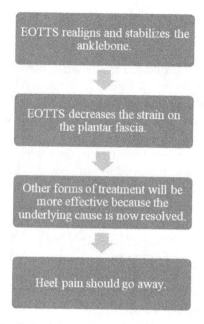

Figure 34. Rationale for the recommendation of EOTTS, when indicated.

There are older, more aggressive, methods of realigning and stabilizing the anklebone. These procedures involve the cutting and shifting of the back of the heel bone, cutting the front of the heel bone, and inserting bone grafts—and bone grafts just fuse the anklebone and heel bone. There are also other soft-tissue procedures, as were discussed in a previous chapter, but these have not been proven to be best in the long term.

All the traditional surgical procedures involve lengthy surgery times and long recoveries, and they have many associated risks and complications. For example, many patients have to go back to the operating room later to have painful pins and screws removed or to have revision surgery. This irreversible bone surgery is usually reserved for severe, end-stage foot alignment treatment.

The EOTTS procedure, however, is brief. A small incision is made below the outer anklebone. Trial sizing is done to determine which size of stent will maintain anklebone alignment while allowing the natural motions to occur, and then the stent is simply pushed into place. It is not screwed or drilled into the bone. Patients are able to walk immediately after the procedure, though they should keep their walking to a minimum for several days to allow the tissues to heal after incision.

Unfortunately, many foot specialists are not truly familiar with the EOTTS procedure. Many different devices have been approved to treat heel pain, causing many doctors to be leery of devices, and because of the bad track record of the type I (arthroereisis) devices used in EOTTS, many doctors have not fully embraced EOTTS as an option. The success of the type II (HyProCure) sinus tarsi implant, however, has made EOTTS more successful. The results are undeniable, and it makes total sense.

How can we realign and stabilize the anklebone on the hindfoot?

As we've already seen (figure 34), arch supports and foot orthotics can't do it! Traditional surgery can, but it's typically much too aggressive. EOTTS makes sense and is scientifically proven to realign and stabilize the anklebone. EOTTS is the only solution proven to decrease the strain on the plantar fascia by 33 percent.[220]

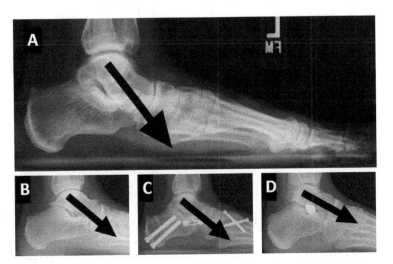

Figure 35. (A) A displaced anklebone. (B) An arch support failing to realign and stabilize the anklebone. (C) An aggressive form of treatment. (D) A sinus tarsi implant internally realigning and stabilizing the anklebone.

You must decide if the treatment you've been prescribed addresses the underlying cause of your problem or is only aimed at the secondary effect: the pain (figure 35). I've written this many times in this book because it is so important, but here it is again: Treatment **must** begin with fixing the *underlying cause*. Otherwise, the symptoms (heel pain, in this case) will keep occurring.

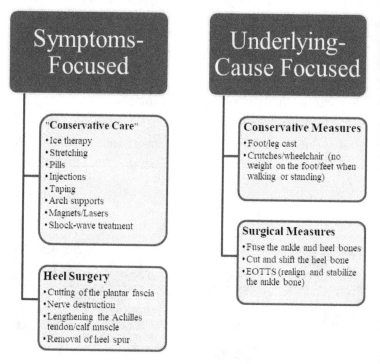

Figure 36. Comparison of heel pain treatments.

Patient Expectation of EOTTS Procedure

The EOTTS procedure takes about fifteen minutes to perform, but the recovery period will be much longer. Each patient and each foot will recover at different rates. Some patients have little to no pain, whereas other patients could take months to even a year or longer for their hindfoot to adjust to the new foot position. There are many factors that can delay the healing process, such as pain tolerance, activity level, ability to heal the post-procedure local inflammation, and the degree of deformity. The ankle and heel bones will instantly be realigned, however, and there will be decreased strain to the plantar fascia.

Most patients will need to have both feet internally stabilized with the EOTTS procedure. It is recommended that patients have one foot stabilized at a time, rather than both at the same surgical setting. This gives the patient one "good" foot to walk on while the other foot heals. But you must be warned that the foot that underwent the EOTTS procedure will continue to have soreness until the opposite foot is also corrected with the EOTTS procedure. It is my experience that having one foot operated on at a time gives patients a fast recovery than having both feet operated on at the same time.

Most patients are able to bear full weight on the foot during the initial recovery period. Some surgeons will prescribe crutches or even a walking brace to assist in the healing process. Most patients are back to fairly normal walking within a few weeks and allowed to run or jog by six to eight weeks, assuming an uneventful recovery.

How soon the heel pain should disappear after the EOTTS procedure is a very important question. This depends on the degree of plantar fascia tissue damage. The more damage and the longer the nerves have been damaged, we would expect it would take longer for those tissues to heal. Some patients have claimed that their heel pain resolved within a few weeks, whereas other patients required more advanced treatments to assist in the healing of the diseased plantar fascial tissue.

There are no guarantees that EOTTS is going to cure, whether in the present or permanently, your heel pain. But you have already learned that failure to address the underlying etiology—a misaligned hindfoot—will compromise the long-term effect of any other form of treatment.

Every solution has the potential of creating a new problem. Look at all the side effects associated with prescription medicine. It's enough to scare you away from taking the medicine. We don't want the cure to be worse than the disease we're trying to treat. EOTTS is a very powerful orthopedic soft-tissue procedure, but there are potential risks with any surgical procedure.

Specific risks associated with EOTTS include displacement or loosening of the stent, partial loss of correction, prolonged pain in the area of the surgery, the need to insert a smaller- or larger-sized stent, the need to permanently remove the stent, prolonged recovery time, and a period of abnormal walking due to the realignment of the hindfoot bones. The potential risks of EOTTS, however, far outweigh the potential risks associated with other surgical procedures to realign and stabilize the hindfoot bones (figure 36).

After reading all of the preceding material, you will have discovered that EOTTS makes the most sense over any other treatment discussed. I truly hope that your heel pain can be resolved without having to have surgery. I also hope that if nonsurgical measures fail to give you the relief you need, you are given the choice to have the EOTTS procedure before a more radical procedure, such as permanently cutting the plantar fascia or fusing other important joints of your foot.

	EOTTS	Heel Bone Cutting/Shifting	Anklebone to heelbone fusion
Decreases strain on the plantar fascia	✓	✓	✓
Can be reversed	✓		
Typically involves second surgery to removal painful screws, pins, staples, or wires.		✓	✓
Less likely to require a second surgery to remove implant	✓		
Is associated with the formation of arthritis in adjacent joints			✓
Proven to stabilize forces between ankle and heel bones.	✓		✓
Inability to stabilize the forces between the ankle and heel bones		✓	
Typically takes < 20 minutes to perform	✓		
Longer surgery and recovery time		✓	✓

Figure 37. Comparison of methods to realign and stabilize the hindfoot.

Develop an Action Plan and Implement It

Chronic heel pain is not a life-and-death condition. It can, however, severely affect your quality of life. As we have seen throughout this book, this is usually a very challenging condition to "cure." There's never been a quick fix, because the focus of attention has been to relieve pain instead of eliminating the underlying cause. The majority of the medical community continues to treat chronic heel pain by trying to resolve an inflammatory condition of the plantar fascia, which, of course, is not the root of the problem. Meanwhile, the mechanical overloading of this tissue continues when patients stand and with every step they take, until the fascia ruptures on its own or a surgeon takes a scalpel to it—though it's a structure that need not be cut.

Unfortunately, as I'm sure you will remember, the story doesn't end there. The excessive abnormal forces that occur as a result of the anklebone's partial dislocation will continue to exert/inflict damage to other parts of the foot and can also wreak havoc up the body to other bodily structures by affecting the alignment of the knees, hips, pelvis, and back. While it is important to end the pain, it is more important to eliminate pain by eliminating the *underlying etiology*. The best way to accomplish this is by stabilizing the actual anklebone dislocation deformity. For this, EOTTS has been shown to be the most effective form of treatment.

Refuse to let your feet slow you down. Take back your quality of life. Find a foot specialist near you who performs the EOTTS procedure to see if EOTTS is the very solution you have been waiting for. Not only will your feet thank you, but so will the rest of your body.

With that said, remember that the majority of foot-care specialists would rather treat the nonexistent inflammation than realign and stabilize the anklebone. It is in your best interest to find a doctor who is interested in fixing the underlying cause while also addressing the symptoms.

It is rare for one treatment to fix many things, especially when it pertains to the foot and ankle. There could be many co-determining factors that lead to the overstretching of the plantar fascia. It may take an assortment of treatments to fix your heel pain. I'm not claiming that if you have a stent placed below your anklebone, your heel pain will magically go away the next day. There are damaged tissues that have to be repaired. While many patients have noticed an immediate improvement in their heel pain, this is not the norm. The real determining factor is how much damage has occurred to the tissues and how fast your body is able to repair that damage.

Don't delay—seek guidance today.

Good luck!

Resources

Here are a few great online sites that will help provide the reader with more information regarding a misaligned hindfoot and the EOTTS solution.

www.AlignMyFeet.com
www.Hyperpronation.com

Glossary

Achilles tendon: Tendon at the back of the heel that extends up to and connects with the calf muscle.

acupuncture: An ancient therapy sometimes used in modern healthcare that utilizes specialized needles.

activity-limiting pain: Pain that is so severe it limits the activity level of the person. The person fears the pain they'll experience because of being active, so they don't perform that activity.

acute: Early in onset, still lingering in its explosiveness, and impactful in magnitude. In regard to heel pain, < 3-month history of pain.

anatomic neck: From the end of a long bone, this very specific region includes the very beginning of the narrower shaft-like middle portion of that bone—the area between the head and body of that bone.

anklebone: Talus; the bone that sits directly atop the heel bone. This bone is extremely relevant to exactly where and how motion occurs to the remainder of the foot and lower limb.

arthritis: Inflammation of at least one joint. Often misnamed to depict general pain or aging of one or more joints.

arthroereisis: A procedure to limit joint motion.

auto-rupture: Breakage that occurs to a structure (such as the plantar fascia) on its own, without surgical intervention. Auto-rupture is often an unfortunate ultimate consequence of prolonged weakness/progression of the structure.

biomechanics: The study or understanding of standard body mechanics/movement/function to a specific or general area. This study appreciates the common interrelationships between musculoskel-etal structures.

bisection: The result of bisecting a structure. Bisection allows better aim or usage of a line of direction of a given bone.

bone spur: Calcium deposit on a bone; a small protuberance of bone at the surface of bone that was acquired over time and is thus not representative of normal or original anatomy.

bone tumor: Growth of bone, either benign or malignant.

bunion: A boney bump on the inside of the big toe joint, often in the presence of a big toe whose alignment angulates toward the adjacent second toe.

calcaneal inclination angle: The angulation that the calcaneus takes against the flat ground surface. Its magnitude correlates directly with the height of the arch and, in effect, causes the arch to be higher.

calcaneus: The heel bone, the largest bone of the foot.

callus: An increased thickening of tissue; most often refers to the skin and is an occurrence that is often reacting to something.

center point of pain: This is the bull's-eye location of pain.

central band of the plantar fascia: The middle elongated section of the plantar fascia. This structure often experiences the greatest amount of pull, as the lower arch structure is so often being stressed or has direct tension applied to it.

chronic: Opposite of acute; a condition that has been present three months or longer.

clinician: A practicing professional working in a clinical setting (versus at a surgical or other location); often refers to a doctor.

comorbidity: Damage that happens at the same time as damage caused by another condition.

contract (as in *contraction*): Reversible shrinking with a clear purpose, as in enabling a muscle (as in foot muscles, heart, etc.) to thus move bones through that very shrinkage.

corticosteroid: A steroid that mimics the steroid(s) produced by the body. Often injected or consumed as a pill or topical medicine.

cryosurgery: Surgery using extreme cold.

curative: Able to, and with a tendency to, cure.

cyma line: A snake-like or S-like curvature of a line, as seen radiographically in the midfoot. It represents the degree of arch stability or a breakdown in arch stability when also seen with arch flatness or breakdown. Pronation will alter this line as well.

dislocation: When referring to a joint, indicates that the joint is misaligned to an extreme degree.

displacement: Two structures positioned out of alignment to a somewhat lesser degree than dislocation would be, and often occurring as a slight sliding out of alignment in one or more planes.

dorsoplantar (DP) view: A view that aims directly from the top (dorsal aspect) of a foot toward the bottom (plantar aspect) of the foot.

electromagnetic field: In medicine, a strong, applied high-frequency energy produced, controlled, and targeted to produce an intended result.

entrapment: The state of being directly covered and quite altered by some other tissue, as would be a nerve from scar tissue that abnormally encases it at a specific area.

Epsom salt: A mineral salt powder that often gets mixed into a water solution to be used for foot soaking.

excision: Surgical removal.

extended-use pulsed radiofrequency: Sound-wave pulses sent into the tissues by an electronic device worn on the heel.

extracorporeal shock-wave therapy: A treatment that targets (or blasts) high-intensity ultrasonic shock waves at a body part to break something up, as in at the attachment of the plantar fascia to break up its inflammation. This same kind of technology is also used to blast kidney stones.

false negative: The absence of a connection, but one later found to be clearly an incorrect finding.

fasciitis: Inflammation of the fascia.

fibula: The thinner of the two parallel bones making up the lower leg (runs alongside the tibia).

first metatarsal: The bone that directly connects with the big toe and comprises a major portion of the arch and of the foot's function.

forefoot: Roughly speaking, the front third of the foot, including the toes and many of the closest bones connecting to them.

fracture: The medical term for a broken bone. Less often, this term can also refer to cartilage.

fuzzy bone spurs: Bone spurs inside a joint that are diffuse, or less defined. Often, this kind of boney tissue is depicting active bone formation.

gait: The walking pattern or walking style of the human frame.

gait cycle: The studied phases of a human's walking pattern that have been well-outlined and labeled as a pattern seen to be clearly repetitious, or cyclic, as one walks.

hammertoe: A curled toe that basically isn't lying in a normal alignment and is buckled, often causing problems in being so.

heel spur: A bone spur to the calcaneus, or heel bone. Seen to be located at the bottom of the bone, versus ones that can often be seen at the back of the heel bone, which are *not* correctly referred to as "heel spurs." Heel spurs are often found in the presence of plantar fasciitis (or plantar fasciosis), though not always.

hindfoot: The back one-third of the foot, connecting directly to the ankle. This area determines much of the foot's overall motion, as this region is essentially where the foot's primary motion derives.

histologic: Referring to the microscopic anatomy of tissues, typically requiring sophisticated and very close observation and examination of that tissue.

immobilization: Locking a body structure so efficiently that no movement can occur to that body part in any fashion—it will not and cannot move.

impingement: The act of interfering or cutting off without severing.

inflammation: The collective and analogous "firelike" effect from tissues. The combined presence of any combination of these factors: redness, swelling, pain, tenderness, and warmth.

inner column of the foot: A row of connecting bones of the foot that connect the inner portion of the midfoot with the inner portion of the forefoot. This involves a few bones and comprises a major portion of the arch as well.

-itis: Found at the end of the name of a structure to indicate that the structure is inflamed.

joint: Where one bone connects to another. In many cases, this kind of connection represents a gap, complete with a sophisticated and slippery structure enabling normal movement of one area of the body against another.

ligament: Strong connective tissue connecting bone to bone.

locking: When one bone is temporarily positioned such that it disallows the movement of others.

low-Dye taping: Taping of the arch in a manner that intentionally controls excessive and problematic movement (or pronation) of the foot and its arches.

low-level laser: A focused light beam that targets a particular body region so as to provide tissue disruption in the area. The intention is for an increased resultant amount of blood supply for that area and for subsequent healing of a specific problematic region.

meta-analysis: An investigation that studies varied methods. As used in this book, it refers to a recent medical investigation studying various methods of realigning the foot, such as motion-control footwear, arch supports, and low-Dye taping/strapping.

metatarsalgia: Pain in the ball of the foot; has various forms and causes.

micro-rupture: A rupture that is harder to detect and of lesser severity than a full rupture.

micro-tear: Same as micro-rupture, though with the perception, or additional component, of tissue stretching.

micro-trauma: Trauma on a small, even microscopic level. Leads to a greater result, or greater tissue damage, if allowed to progress.

midfoot: The approximate middle third of the foot, including various bones and joints in that area.

misaligned: Not properly aligned, enabling abnormal or excessive motion to result from a certain level of structural instability.

misaligned hindfoot: Where the anklebone is tilted from an optimal alignment atop the heel bone, thus enabling a dislocation to that connection and a whole host of subsequent or related foot/leg problems as a result of the abnormal forces from that loss of proper alignment.

mobile adapter: The foot's display of "softening" in its movement so as to effectively conform to various uneven surfaces while absorbing forces/shock and, thus, retain balance and a normal foot function. Foot pronation enables this display.

MRI: Magnetic resonance imaging; a sophisticated image of the anatomy made by utilizing magnetics to create a more detailed identification of various problems contained within the targeted tissues. This is not an X-ray.

navicular: A bone in the foot that is part of the arch, integral in many ways to proper foot movement. It connects on one side to the anklebone and on the other end to smaller (cuneiform) bones of the midfoot.

nerve fibers: Multiple small nerves connected in one area.

neuropathy: A disease of the nerves that alters nerve function. Both pain and numbness can be associated with neuropathy.

night splint: A device worn at night to help immobilize a body part to a degree. A very common night splint is used to help manage plantar fasciitis/fasciosis at times.

non-weightbearing: Describing a position in which the body or a particular body part does not bear weight against the ground surface.

orthotic: With the foot, this term often refers to a conforming device placed under one's foot.

-osis: used at the end of the name of a structure or system to indicate that the structure or system is problematic.

osseous: Referring to bone.

overloading (as with the bones of the inner foot): Undesired and abnormal stresses of weightbearing forces on one area.

paratenon: The normal outer covering of many tendons.

pathological: On a basic level, this refers to the idea of "causing problems" or that it is clearly able to.

pathology: In the body, this term simply represents a problem or the progression *toward* a disorder or problem.

periosteum: The tissue membrane on the surface of all bones.

plantar fascia release: Surgical cutting of the plantar fascia.

plantar fasciitis: Inflammation of the plantar fascia, which is, technically, relatively rare. The term is overused, typically inaccurately.

plantar fasciopathy: Essentially means that there is something wrong with the plantar fascia—generically or otherwise.

plantar fasciosis: A tearing degeneration of the plantar fascia due to mechanical overloading forces.

plantar fasciotomy: Surgical severing of the plantar fascia, usually at its direct connection to the heel bone.

platelet-rich plasma (PRP): A solution containing healing cells originally drawn from a patient's blood. The substance is then injected back into the body, at or near specific areas of need.

posterior tibial tendon: The stabilizing tendon at the arch of the foot that helps maintain the arch and directly connects the posterior tibial muscle to the arch bones for proper foot support and function.

pronation: An oblique, diagonal direction of movement of the foot (or hand) that is in opposite direction of supination. In its relevance to normal foot function, pronation needs to occur (though not in excess), as a proper amount of pronation enables a necessary degree of shock-absorption function to take place and allows the foot and leg to adapt to various surfaces, utilizing surface adaptation.

radio-frequency nerve ablation: A treatment that involves insertion of an electrical probe into deep tissue in order to send an electrical impulse to the tissue to shut down the nerve and deaden pain.

radiograph: An X-ray view; an X-ray film.

radiographic: Pertaining to a radiograph, its findings, or an X-ray.

range of motion: The full motion of a joint, often measured in total degrees.

rule out: To determine something as not being a possibility.

rupture: A complete snapping, popping, or bursting of a tissue or organ.

second metatarsal: A long bone of the forefoot that connects to the bones of the second toe. Its "head" makes up a portion of the ball of the foot. This bone is somewhat less integral to the arch than is the first metatarsal.

silicone: A lab-made nylon polymer that is a rather soft, clear material containing both polyester and silicon; often used as the primary substance for various bodily implants.

sinus tarsi/sinus tarsi space: The normal cavity, or space, of the hindfoot. The small region of the hindfoot where the anklebone lies directly atop and moves upon the heel bone. This is exactly where the main shock-absorbing motion of the entire leg directly derives.

sinus tarsi stent: A medical implant placed into the sinus tarsi.

soft tissue: All tissue in the body, aside from bone and cartilage.

stance phase: The momentary part of the gait cycle where the foot is in complete contact with the ground. It represents the phase of gait that is directly opposite the swing phase.

stent: Medical implant that is inserted into a naturally occurring space.

steroid: See *corticosteroid*.

strain: The painful effect on a specific structure that has had direct stress, pull, or tension applied to it, with a subsequent need to have to heal that effect.

strapping: See *low-Dye taping*.

stress fracture: A fracture of bone that is often difficult to see on an X-ray and can get missed. It often occurs from repeated stresses onto that bone over time, versus from traumatic impact. Often referred to as a "march fracture" or "fatigue fracture."

supination: Opposite of pronation. Allows for propulsion of gait by making the foot a rigid lever. Supination can be a movement or a position of the foot that derives from hindfoot action.

surgical rupture: A rupture to a structure that occurred directly *through* a surgical procedure.

swing phase: The momentary part of the gait cycle where the foot is completely off of the ground as it is moving. It represents the phase of gait that is directly opposite to the stance phase. The foot and leg are, in essence, "swinging" forward to be able to ultimately reach the ground.

symptom: As opposed to a "sign," this is basically what a patient *feels* and is not necessarily noticed visually or by measurement.

talar-second metatarsal angle: An angle drawn from measuring the bisection (or pointing) of the anklebone (talus) against that of the second metatarsal. It represents foot position and a degree of foot stability.

talotarsal: Referring to the joints connecting the anklebone (talus) to both the heel bone (calcaneus) and the navicular (arch bone).

talus: Anklebone.

tendon: Strong connective tissue connecting muscle to bone.

tibia: The thicker of the two parallel bones making up the lower leg (runs alongside the fibula). Connects directly to the anklebone.

tissue: The simple "substance" of the body in general, in all its varied forms and locations. Excludes the fluids, sheddings, or excretions of the body.

trauma: Physical action against the body that causes damage, destruction, pain, discomfort, or harm in some way.

ultrasonic imaging: In directly using sound waves to do so, a picture is created that can be directly viewed. This can be a still image or a video. It is not an X-ray.

ultrasound: Sound waves of a particular frequency. This frequency is in the inaudible range. It can be used to capture an actual image— even toward a diagnosis. It can also be used therapeutically to certain areas of the body in order to treat a problem or ailment.

vascularity: The status of one's blood supply and blood vessels, including arteries as well as veins, along with their smallest versions (i.e., capillaries, venues, valves, etc.).

weightbearing: Describing a position in which the body or a particular body part bears direct weight against the ground surface.

Endnotes

Chapter 1

1. Tong KB, Furia J. Economic burden of plantar fasciitis treatment in the United States. Am J Orthop (Belle Mead NJ). May;39(5):227–31, 2010.

2. Graham ME, Jawrani NT, Goel VK. Evaluating plantar fascia strain in hyperpronating cadaveric feet following an extra-osseous talotarsal stabilization procedure. J Foot Ankle Surg. 50(6):682–6, 2011.

3. Cheung JT, Zhang M, An KN. Effects of plantar fascia stiffness on the biomechanical responses of the ankle-foot complex. Clin Biomech (Bristol Avon). 19(8):839–46, 2004.

4. van de Water AT, Speksnijder CM. Efficacy of taping for the treatment of plantar fasciosis: a systematic review of controlled trials. J Am Podiatr Med Assoc. 100(1):41–51, 2010.

5. Cheung JT, An KN, Zhang M. Consequences of partial and total plantar fascia release: a finite element study. Foot Ankle Int. 27(2):125–32, 2006.

6. Cheung JT, Zhang M, An KN. Effects of plantar fascia stiffness on the biomechanical responses of ankle-foot complex. Clin Biomech (Bristol, Avon). 19(8):839–46, 2004.

7. Crary JL, Hollis JM, Manoli A 2nd. The effect of plantar fascia release on strain in the spring and long plantar ligaments. Foot Ankle Int. 24(3):245–50, 2003.

8. Gibbs RC, Boxer MC. Abnormal biomechanics of feet and their cause of hyperkeratoses. J Am Acad Dermatol. 1982;6(6):1061–9.

9. Nubé VL, Molyneaux L, Yue DK. Biomechanical risk factors associated with neuropathic ulceration of the hallux in people with diabetes mellitus. J Am Podiatr Med Assoc. 2006;96(3):189–97.

10. Rao S, Song J, Kraszewski A, Backus S, Ellis SJ, Deland JT, et al. The effect of foot structure on the 1st metatarsophalangeal joint flexibility and hallucal loading. Gait Posture. 2011;34(1):131–7.

Chapter 2

11. Sheridan L, Lopez A, Perez A, John MM, Willis FB, Shanmugam R. Plantar fasciopathy treated with dynamic splinting: a randomized controlled trial. J Am Podiatr Med Assoc. 100(3):161–5, 2010.

12. Tone KB, Furia J. Economic burden of plantar fasciitis treatment in the United States. Am J Orthop. 39(5):227–231, 2010.

13. Crawford F, Thomson C. Interventions for treating plantar heel pain. Cochrane Database Syst. Rev. 3:CD000416, 2003.

14. Nyasani E, Munir I, Perez M, Payne K, Khan S. Linking obesity-induced leptin-signaling pathways to common endocrine-related cancers in women. Endocrine. 2019 Jan;63(1):3–17.

15. Lengyel E, Makowski L, DiGiovanni J, Kolonin MG. Cancer as a Matter of Fat: The Crosstalk between Adipose Tissue and Tumors. Trends Cancer. 2018 May;4(5):374–384.

16. Martin JE, Hosch JC, Goforth WP, Murff RT, Lynch DM, Odom RD. Mechanical treatment of plantar fasciitis. A prospective study. J Am Podiatr Med Assoc. 91(2):55–62, 2001.

17. Salvioli S, Guidi M, Marcotulli G. The effectiveness of conservative, non-pharmacological treatment, of plantar heel pain: a systematic review with meta-analysis. Foot(Edinb). 33:57–67, 2017.

18. Mischke JJ, Javaseelan DJ, Sault JD, Emerson Kavchak AJ. The symptomatic and functional effects of manual physical therapy on plantar heel pain: a systematic review. J Man Manip Ther. 25(1):3–10, 2017.

19. Rompe JD, Furia J, Weil L, Maffulli N. Shock wave therapy for chronic plantar fasciopathy. Br Med Bull. 81(82):183–208, 2007.

Chapter 3

20. Chen DW, Li B, Aubeeluck A, Yang YF, Huang YG, Zhou JQ, Yu GR. Anatomy and biomechanical properties of the plantar aponeurosis: a cadaveric study. PLoS One. 9(1):e84347, 2014.

21. Stecco C, Corradin M, Macchi V, Morra A, Porzionato A, Biz C, De Caro R. Plantar fascia anatomy and its relationship with Achilles tendon and paratenon. J Atom. 223(6):665–76, 2013.

22. Stecco C, Corradin M, Macchi V, Morra A, Porzionato A, Biz C, De Caro R. Plantar fascia anatomy and its relationship with Achilles tendon and paratenon. J Anat. 223(6):665–76, 2013.

23. Thordarson DB, Schmotzer H, Chon J, Peters J. Dynamic support of the human longitudinal arch: a biomechanical evaluation. Clin Orthop. 316:165–72, 1995.

24. Kitaoka HB, Luo ZP, Growney ES, Berglund LJ, An KN. Material properties of the plantar aponeurosis. Foot Ankle Int. 15(10):557–60, 1994.

25. Caravaggi P, Pataky T, Gunther M, Savage R, Crompton R. Dynamics of longitudinal arch support in relation to walking speed: contribution of the plantar aponeurosis. J Anat. 217(3):254–61, 2010.

26. Pavan PG, Stecco C, Darwish S, Natali AN, De Caro R. Investigation of the mechanical properties of the plantar aponeurosis. Surg Radiol Anat. 33(10):905–11, 2011.

27. Cheung JT, Zang M, An KN. Effects of plantar fascia stiffness on the biomechanical responses of ankle-foot complex. Clin Biomech (Bristol, Avon). 19(8):839–46, 2004.

28. Cralley JC, Schuberth JM, Fitch KL. The deep band of the plantar aponeurosis of the human foot. Anat Anz. 152(2):189–97, 1982.

29. Bojsen-Moller F, Flagstad KE. Plantar aponeurosis and internal architecture of the ball of the foot. J Anat. 121(Pt 3)599–6111, 1976.

30. Caravaggi P, Pataky T, Goulemans JY, Savage R, Crompton R. A dynamic model of the windlass mechanism of the foot: evidence for early stance phase preloading of the plantar aponeurosis. J Exp Biol. 212(Pt 15):249–9, 2009.

31. Erdemir A, Hamel AJ, Fauth AR, Piazza SJ, Sharkey NA. Dynamic loading of the plantar aponeurosis in walking. J Bone Joint Surg Am. 86-A(3):546–52, 2004.

32. Fessel G, Jacob HA, Wyss CH, Mittimeier T, Muller-Gerbl M, Buttner A. Changes in length of the plantar aponeurosis during the stance phase of gait—an in vivo dynamic fluoroscopic study. Ann Anat. 196(6):471–8, 2014.

33. Chen H, Ho HM, Ying M, Fu SN. Association between plantar fascia vascularity and morphology and foot dysfunction in individuals with chronic plantar fasciitis. J Orthop Sports Phys Ther. 43(10):727–34, 2013.

34. Chandler TJ, Kibler WB. A biomechanical approach to the prevention, treatment and rehabilitation of plantar fasciitis. Sports Med. 15(5):344–52, 1993.

35. Wolgin M, Cook C, Graham C, Mauldin D. Conservative treatment of plantar heel pain: long-term follow-up. Foot Ankle Int. 15(3):97–102, 1994.

Chapter 6

36. Graham M, Chikka A, Jones P. Validation of the Talar–Second Metatarsal Angle as a Standard Measurement for Radiographic Evaluation. J Am Podiatr Med Assoc. 101(5):390–9, 2011.

37. Mohseni-Bandpei MA, Makhaee M, Mousavi ME, Shakourirad A, Safari MR, Vahab Kashani R. Application of ultrasound in the assessment of plantar fascia in patients with plantar fasciitis: a systematic review. Ultrasound Med Biol. 40(8):1737–54, 2014.

38. Abul K, Ozer D, Sakizlioglu SS, Buyuk AF, Kaygusuz MA. Detection of normal plantar fascia thickness in adults via the ultrasonographic method. J Am Podiatr Med Assoc. 105(1):8–13, 2015.

39. McNally EG, Shetty S. Plantar fascia: imaging diagnosis and guided treatment. Semin Musculoskeletal Radiol. 14(3):334–43, 2010.

40. Fabrikant JM, Park TS. Plantar fasciitis (fasciosis) treatment outcome study: plantar fascia thickness measured by ultrasound and correlated with patient self-reported improvement. Foot (Edinb). 21(2):79–83, 2011.

41. Gadalla N, Kichouh M, Boulet C, Machiels F, De Mey J, De Maeseneer M. Sonographic evaluation of the plantar fascia in asymptomatic subjects. JBR-BTR. 97(5):271–3, 2014.

42. Zhang L, Wan W. Zhang L, Xiao H, Lou Y, Fei X, Zheng Z, Tang P. Assessment of plantar fasciitis using shear wave elastography. Nan Fang Yi Ke Da Xue Xue Bao. 34(2):206–9, 2014.

Chapter 7

43. Ribeiro AP, Joao SM, Dinato RC, Tessutti VD, Sacco IC. Dynamic patterns of forces and loading rate in runners with unilateral plantar fasciitis: a cross-sectional study. PLoS One. 10(9):e0136971, 2015.

44. Golightly YM, Hannan MT, Dufour AB, Hillstrom HJ, Jordan JM. Foot disorders associated with overpronated and oversupinated foot function: the Johnston County osteoarthritis project. Foot Ankle Int. 35(11):1159–65, 2014.

45. Chang R, Rodriques PA, Van Emmerik RE, Hamill J. Multi-segment foot kinematics and ground reaction forces during gait of individuals with plantar fasciitis. J Biomech. 47(11):2571–7, 2014.

46. Graham ME, Jawrani NT, Goel VK. Evaluating plantar fascia strain in hyperpronating cadaveric feet following an extra-osseous talotarsal stabilization procedure. J Foot Ankle Surg. 50(6):682–6, 2011.

47. Caravaggi P, Pataky T, Gunther M, Savage R, Cromptom R. Dynamics of longitudinal arch support in relation to walking speed: contribution of the plantar aponeurosis. J Aat. 217(3):254–61, 2010.

48. Lee Sy, Hertel J, Lee SC. Rearfoot eversion has indirect effects on plantar fascia tension by changing the amount of arch collapse. Foot (Edinb). 20(2–3):64–70, 2010.

49. Hammer WI. The effect of mechanical load on degenerated soft tissue. J Body Mov Ther. 12(3):246–56, 2008.

50. Erdemir A, Hamel AJ, Fauth AR, Piazza SJ, Sharkey NA. Dynamic loading of the plantar aponeurosis in walking. J Bone Joint Surg Am. 86-A(3):546–52, 2004.

51. Bolgla LA, Malone TR. Plantar fasciitis and the windlass mechanism: a biomechanical link to clinical practice. J Athl Train. 39(1):77–82, 2004.

52. Cheung JT, Zhang M, An KN. Effects of plantar fascia stiffness on the biomechanical responses of the ankle-foot complex. Clin Biomech (Bristol Avon). 19(8):839–46, 2004.

53. Gafen A. The in vivo elastic properties of the plantar fascia during the contact phase of walking. Foot Ankle Int. 24(3):238–44, 2003.

54. Kwong PK, Kay D, Vorner RT, White MW. Plantar fasciitis: mechanics and pathomechanics of treatment. Clin Sports Med. 7(1):119–26, 1988.

55. Sarrafian SK. Functional characteristics of the foot and plantar aponeurosis under tibiotalar loading. Foot Ankle. 8(1):4–18, 1987.

56. Purcell RL, Schroeder IG, Keeling LE, Formby PM, Eckel TT, Shawen SB. Clinical Outcomes After Extracorporeal Shock Wave Therapy for Chronic Plantar Fasciitis in a Predominantly Active Duty Population. J Foot Ankle Surg. 2018 Jul-Aug;57(4):654–657.

57. Yi TI, Lee GE, Seo IS, Huh WS, Yoon TH, Kim BR. Clinical characteristics of the causes of plantar heel pain. Ann Rehabil Med. 2011 Aug;35(4):507–13.

Chapter 8

58. Lemont H, Ammirati KM, Usen N. Plantar fasciitis: a degenerative process (fasciosis) without inflammation. J Am Pod Med Assoc. 93(3):2347, 2003.

59. Schepsis AA, Leach RE, Gorzyca J. Plantar fasciitis: etiology, treatment, surgical results, and review of the literature. Clin Orthop. 266:185–96, 1991.

60. Tountas AA, Fornasier I. Operative treatment of subcalcaneal pain. Clin Orthop. 332:170–8, 1996.

61. Karls SL, Snyder KR, Neibert PJ. Effectiveness of corticosteroid injections in the treatment of plantar fasciosis. J Sport Rehabil. 25(2):202–7, 2016.

62. Wearing SC, Smeathers JE, Urry SR, Henning EM, Hills AP. The pathomechanics of plantar fasciitis. Sports Med. 36(7):585–611, 2006.

63. Ribeiro AP, Joao SM, Dinato RC, Tessutti VD, Sacco IC. Dynamic patterns of forces and loading rate in runners with unilateral plantar fasciitis: a cross-sectional study. PLoS One. 10(9):e0136971, 2015.

64. Golightly YM, Hannan MT, Dufour AB, Hillstrom HJ, Jordan JM. Foot disorders associated with overpronated and oversupinated foot function: the Johnston County osteoarthritis project. Foot Ankle Int. 35(11):1159–65, 2014.

65. Chang R, Rodriques PA, Van Emmerik RE, Hamill J. Multi-segment foot kinematics and ground reaction forces during gait of individuals with plantar fasciitis. J Biomech. 47(11):2571–7, 2014.

66. Graham ME, Jawrani NT, Goel VK. Evaluating plantar fascia strain in hyperpronating cadaveric feet following an extra-osseous talotarsal stabilization procedure. J Foot Ankle Surg. 50(6):682–6, 2011.

67. Caravaggi P, Pataky T, Gunther M, Savage R, Cromptom R. Dynamics of longitudinal arch support in relation to walking speed: contribution of the plantar aponeurosis. J Aat. 217(3):254–61, 2010.

68. Lee Sy, Hertel J, Lee SC. Rearfoot eversion has indirect effects on plantar fascia tension by changing the amount of arch collapse. Foot (Edinb). 20(2–3):64–70, 2010.

69. Hammer WI. The effect of mechanical load on degenerated soft tissue. J Body Mov Ther. 12(3):246–56, 2008.

70. Erdemir A, Hamel AJ, Fauth AR, Piazza SJ, Sharkey NA. Dynamic loading of the plantar aponeurosis in walking. J Bone Joint Surg Am. 86-A(3):546–52, 2004.

71. Bolgla LA, Malone TR. Plantar fasciitis and the windlass mechanism: a biomechanical link to clinical practice. J Athl Train. 39(1):77–82, 2004.

72. Cheung JT, Zhang M, An KN. Effects of plantar fascia stiffness on the biomechanical responses of the ankle-foot complex. Clin Biomech (Bristol Avon). 19(8):839–46, 2004.

73. Gafen A. The in vivo elastic properties of the plantar fascia during the contact phase of walking. Foot Ankle Int. 24(3):238–44, 2003.

74. Kwong PK, Kay D, Vorner RT, White MW. Plantar fasciitis. Mechanics and pathomechanics of treatment. Clin Sports Med. 7(1):119–26, 1988.

75. Sarrafian SK. Functional characteristics of the foot and plantar aponeurosis under tibiotalar loading. Foot Ankle. 8(1):4–18, 1987.

76. Wearing SC, Smeathers JE, Urry SR, Henning EM, Hills AP. The patho-mechanics of plantar fasciitis. Sports Med. 36(7):585–611, 2006.

77. Huang YC, Wang LY, Wang HC, Chang KL, Leong CP. The relationship between the flexible flatfoot and plantar fasciitis: ultrasonographic evaluation. Chang Gung Med J. 27(6):43–8, 2004.

Chapter 9

78. Sahin N, Ozturk A, Atici T. Foot mobility and plantar fascia elasticity in patients with plantar fasciitis. Acta Orthop Traumatol Turc. 44(5):385–91, 2010.

79. Yi TI, Lee GE, Seo IS, Huh WS, Yoon TH, Kim BR. Clinical character-istics of the causes of plantar heel pain. Ann Rehabil Med. 35(4):507–13, 2011.

80. McPoil T, Cornwall MW. Relationship between neutral subtalar joint position and pattern of rearfoot motion during walking. Foot Ankle Int. 15(3):141–5, 1994.

81. Sarrafian SK. Biomechanics of the subtalar complex. Clin Orthop Relat Res. 290:17–26, 1993.

82. Cheung JT, Zang M, An KN. Effects of plantar fascia stiffness on the biomechanical responses of ankle-foot complex. Clin Biomech (Bristol, Avon). 19(8):839–46, 2004.

83. Gefen A. The in vivo elastic properties of the plantar fascia during the contact phase of walking. Foot Ankle Int. 24(3):238–44, 2003.

84. Perry J. Anatomy and biomechanics of the hindfoot. Clin Orthop Relat Res. 177:9–15, 1983.

85. McDonald KA, Stearne SM, Alderson JA, North I, Pires NJ, Rubenson J. The role of arch compression and metatarsophalangeal joint dynamics in modulating plantar fascia strain in running. PLoS One. 11(4):e015602, 2016.

86. Wager JC, Challis JH. Elastic energy within the human plantar aponeu-rosis contributes to arch shortening during the push-off phase of running. J Biomech. 49(5):704–9, 2016.

87. Green SM, Briggs PJ. Flexion strength of the toes in the normal foot. An evaluation using magnetic resonance imaging. Foot (Edinb). 23(4):115–9, 2013.

88. Sarrafian SK. Functional characteristics of the foot and plantar aponeurosis under tibiotalar loading. Foot Ankle. 8(1):4–18, 1987.

89. Lin SC, Chen CP, Tang SF, Wong AM, Hsieh JH, Chen WP. Changes in windlass effect in response to different shoe and insole designs during walking. Gait Posture. 37(2):235–41, 2013.

90. Vereecke EE, Aerts P. The mechanics of the gibbon foot and its potential for elastic energy storage during bipedalism. J Exp Biol. 211(Pt 23):3661–70, 2008.

91. Stokes IAF, Hutton WC, Stott JR. Forces acting on the metatarsal during normal walking. J Anat. 129(Pt #):579–90, 1979.

92. Graham ME, Jawrani NT, Goel VK. Evaluating plantar fascia strain in hyperpronating cadaveric feet following an extra-osseous talotarsal stabilization procedure. J Foot Ankle Surg. 50(6):682–6, 2011.

93. Bolgla LA, Malone TR. Plantar fasciitis and the windlass mechanism: a biomechanical link to clinical practice. J Athl Train. 39(1):77–82, 2004.

94. Carlson RE, Fleming LL, Hutton WC. The biomechanical relationship between the tendoachilles, plantar fascia and metatarsophalangeal joint dorsiflexion angle. Foot Ankle Int. 21(1):18–25, 2000.

95. Donahue SW, Sharkey NA. Strains in the metatarsals during the stance phase of gait: implications for stress fractures. J Bone Joint Surg Am. 81(9):1236–44, 1999.

96. Thordarson DB, Schmotzer H, Chon J, Peters J. Dynamic support of the human longitudinal arch. A biomechanical evaluation. Clin Orthop Relat Res. 316:165–72, 1995.

Chapter 10

97. Baxter DE, Thigpen CM. Heel pain-operative results. Foot Ankle. 5(1):16–25, 1984.

98. Alshami AM, Souvlis T, Coppieters MW. A review of plantar heel pain of neural origin: differential diagnosis and management. Man Ther. 13(2):103–11, 2008.

99. Chen H, Ho HM, Ying M, Fu SN. Association between plantar fascia vascularity and morphology and foot dysfunction in indivuduals with chronic plantar fasciitis. J Orthop Sports Phys Ther. 43(10):727–34, 2013.

100. Didia BC, Horsefall AU. Medial calcaneal nerve: An anatomical study. J Am Podiatr Med Assoc. 80(3):115–9, 1990.

101. Govsa F, Bilge O, Ozer MA. Variations in the origin of the medial and inferior calcaneal nerves. Arch Orthop Trauma Surg. 126(1):6–14, 2006.

102. Louisia S, Masquelet AC. The medial and inferior calcaneal nerves: an anatomic study. Surg Radiol Anat. 21(3):169–73, 1999.

103. Schon LC, Glennon P, Baxter DE. Heel pain syndrome: electrodiagnostic support for nerve entrapment. Foot Ankle. 14(3):129–35, 1993.

104. Chundru U, Liebeskind A, Seidelmann F, Fogel J, Franklin P, Beltran J. Plantar fasciitis and calcaneal spur formation are associated with abductor digiti minimi atrophy on MRI of the foot. Skeletal Radiol. 37(6):505–10, 2008.

105. Rodriques RN, Lopes AA, Torres JM, Mundim MF, Silva LL, Silva BR. Compressive neuropathy of the first branch of the lateral plantar nerve: a study by magnetic resonance imaging. Radiol Bras. 48(6):368–72, 2015.

106. Dirim B, Resnick D, Ozenler NK. Bilateral Baxter's neuropathy secondary to plantar fasciitis. Med Sci Monit. 16(4):CS50–53, 2010.

107. Mizuno D, Naito M, Hayashi S, Ohmichi Y, Ohmichi M, Nakano T. Sex differences in the branching position of the nerve to the abductor digiti minimi muscle: an anatomical study of cadavers. J Foot Ankle Res. 8:22, 2015.

108. Moustafa AM, Hassanein E, Foti C. Objective assessment of corticosteroid effect in plantar fasciitis: additional utility of ultrasound. Muscles Ligaments Tendons J. 59(4):289–96, 2016.

109. Fernandez-Lao C, Galiano-Castillo N, Cantarero-Villanueva I, Martin-Martin L, Prados-Olleta N, Arroyo-Morales M. Analysis of pressure pain hypersensitivity, ultrasound image, and quality of life in patients with chronic plantar pain: a preliminary study. Pain Med. 17(8):1530–41, 2016.

110. Coppieters MW, Alshami AM, Babri AS, Souvlis T, Kippers V, Hodges PW. Strain and excursion of the sciatic, tibial, and plantar nerves during a modified straight leg raising test. J Orthop Res. 24(9):1883–9, 2006.

111. Rondhuis JJ, Huson A. The first branch of the lateral plantar nerve and heel pain. Acta Morphol Neerl Scand. 24(4):269–79, 1986.

Chapter 12

112. Goff JD, Crawford R. Diagnosis and treatment of plantar fasciitis. Am Fam Physician. 84(6):676–82, 2011.

113. Wolgin M, Cook C, Graham C, Mauldin D. Conservative treatment of plantar heel pain: long-term follow up. Foot Ankle Int. 15(3):97–102.

114. Michelsson O, Konttitnen YT, Paavolainen P, Santavirta S. Plantar heel pain and its 3-mode 4-stage treatment. Mod Rheumatol. 15(5):307–14, 2005.

115. Irving DB, Cook JL, Young MA, Menz HB. Impact of chronic plantar heel pain on health-related quality of life. J Am Podiatric Med Assoc. 8(4):283–9, 2008.

116. Lin SC, Chen CP, Tang SF, Wong AM, Hsieh JH, Chen WP. Changes in windlass effect in response to different shoe and insole designs during walking. Gait Posture. 37(2):235–41, 2013.

117. Yu J, Wong DW, Zang H, Lou ZP, Zhang M. The influence of high-heeled shoes on strain and tension force on the anterior talofibular ligament and plantar fascia during balanced standing and walking. Med Eng Phys. 38(10):1152–6, 2016.

118. Kogler GF, Veer FB, Verhulst SJ, Solomonidis SE, Paul JP. The effect of heel elevation on strain within the plantar aponeurosis: in vitro study. Foot Ankle Int. 22(5):433–9, 2001.

119. Solan MC, Carne A, Davies MS. Gastrocnemius shortening and heel pain. Foot Ankle Clin. 19(4):719–38, 2014.

120. Cheng HY, Lin CL, Wang HW, Chou SW. Finite element analysis of the plantar fascia under stretch—the relative contribution of windlass mechanism and Achilles tendon force. J Biomech. 41(9):1937–44, 2008.

121. Cheung JT, Zhang M, An KN. Effect of Achilles tendon loading on plantar fascia tension in the standing foot. Clin Biomech (Bristol, Avon). 21(2):194–203, 2006.

122. Stecco C, Corradin M, Macchi V, Morra A, Porzionato A, Biz C, De Caro R. Plantar fascia anatomy and its relationship with Achilles tendon and paratenon. J Anat. 223(6):665–76, 2013.

123. Rasu RS1, Vouthy K, Crowl AN, Stegeman AE, Fikru B, Bawa WA, Knell ME. Cost of pain medication to treat adult patients with nonmalignant chronic pain in the United States. J Manag Care Spec Pharm. 2014 Sep;20(9):921–8.

124. Donley BG, Moore T, Sferra J, Gozdanovic J, Smith R. The efficacy of oral nonsteroidal anti-inflammatory medication (NSAID) in the treatment of plantar fasciitis: a randomized, prospective, placebo-controlled study. Foot Ankle Int. 28(1):20–3, 2007.

125. Kim C, Cashdollar MR, Mendicino RW, Catanzariti AR, Fuge L. Incidence of plantar fascia ruptures following corticosteroid injection. Foot Ankle Spec. 3(6):335–7, 2010.

126. Kayhan A, Gokay NS, Alpaslan R, Demirok M, Yilmaz J, Gokce A. Sonographically guided corticosteroid injection for the treatment of plantar fasciosis. J Ultrasound Med. 30(4):509–15, 2011.

127. Lemont H, Ammirati KM, Usen N. Plantar fasciitis: a degenerative process (fasciosis) without inflammation. J Am Pod Med Assoc. 93(3):234–7, 2003.

128. Karls SL, Snyder KR, Neibert PJ. Effectiveness of corticosteroid injections in the treatment of plantar fasciosis. J Sport Rehabil. 25(2):202–7, 2016.

129. Guner S, Onder H, Guner SI, Ceylan MG, Goklap MA, Keskin S. Effectiveness of local tenoxicam versus corticosteroid injection for plantar fasciitis. Orthopedics. 36(10):e1322–6, 2013.

130. Lafuente Guijosa A, O'mullony Munoz L, de La Fuente ME, Cura-Ituarte P. Plantar fasciitis: evidence-based review of treatment. Reumatol Clin. 3(4):159–65, 2007.

131. Li Z, Yu A, Qi B, Zhao Y, Wang W, Li P, Ding J. Corticosteroid versus placebo injection for plantar fasciitis: a meta-analysis of randomized controlled trials. Exp Ther Med. 9(6):2263–2268, 2015.

132. Acevedo JI, Beskin JL. Complications of plantar fascia rupture associated with corticosteroid injection. Foot Ankle Int. 19(2):91–7, 1998.

133. Wilson JJ, Lee KS, Miller T, Wang S. Platelet-rich plasma for the treatment of chronic plantar fasciopathy in adults: a case series. 7(1):61–7, 2014.

134. Karls SL, Snyder KR, Neibert PJ. Effectiveness of corticosteroid injections in the treatment of plantar fasciosis. J Sport Rehabil. 25(2):202–7, 2016.

135. van Egmand JC, Breugem SJ, Driessen M, Brulin DJ. Platelet-rich-plasma injection seems to be effective in treatment of plantar fasciitis: a case series. Acta Ortho Belg. 81(2):315–20, 2015.

136. Niazi NS, Hhan Niazi SN, Khan Niazi KN, Igbal M. Effect of the silicone heel pad on plantar fasiciitis. J Pak Med Assoc. 65(11 Suppl):S123–7, 2015.

137. van de Water AT, Speksnijder CM. Efficacy of taping for the treatment of plantar fasciosis: a systematic review of controlled trials. J Am Podiatr Med Assoc. 100(1):41–51, 2010.

138. Lynch DM, Goforth WP, Martin JE, Odom RD, Preece CK, Kotter MW. Conservative treatment of plantar fasciitis: A prospective study. J Am Podiatr Med Assoc. 88(8):375–80, 1998.

139. O'Sullivan K, Kennedy N, O'Neill E, Ni Mhainin U. The effect of low-Dye taping on rearfoot motion and plantar pressure during the stance phase of gait. BMC Musculoskelet Disord. 18(9):111, 2008.

140. Park C, Lee S, Lim DY, Yi CW, Kim JH, Jeon C. Effects of the application of low-Dye taping on the pain and stability of patients. J Phys Ther Sci. 27(8):2491–3, 2015.

141. Deschamps K, Dingenen B, Pans F, Van Bavel I, Matricali GA, Staes F. Effect of taping on foot kinematics in persons with chronic ankle instability. J Sci Med Sport. 19(7):541–6, 2016.

142. Newell T, Simon J, Docherty CL. Arch-taping techniques for altering navicular height and plantar pressures during activity. J Athl Train. 50(8):825–32, 2015.

143. Yoho R, Rivera JJ, Renschler R, Vardaxis VG, Dikis J. A biomechanical analysis of the effects of low-Dye taping on the arch deformation during gait. Foot (Edinb). 22(4):283–6, 2012.

144. Franettovich M, Chapman A, Blanch P, Vicenzino B. Continual use of augmented low-Dye taping increases arch height in standing but does not influence neuromotor control of gait. Gait Posture. 31(2):247–50, 2010.

145. Van Lunen B, Cortes N, Andrus T, Walker M, Pasquale M, Onate J. Immediate effects of a heel-pain orthosis and an augmented low-Dye taping on plantar pressures and pain in subjects with plantar fasciitis. Clin J Sports Med. 21(6):474–9, 2011.

146. Franettovich MM, Murley GS, David BS, Bird AR. A comparison of augmented low-Dye taping and ankle bracing on lower limb muscle activity during walking in adults with flat-arched foot posture. J Sci Med Sport. 15(1):8–13, 2012.

147. Steber S, Kolodziej L. Analysis of radiographic outcomes comparing foot orthosis to extra-osseous talotarsal stabilization in the treatment of recurrent talotarsal joint dislocation. J Min Inv Orthop. 1:1–11, 2015.

148. Kogler GF, Veer FB, Solomonidis SE, Paul JP. The influence of medial and lateral placement of orthotic wedges on loading of the plantar aponeurosis. J Bone Joint Surg Am. 81(10):1403–13, 1999.

149. Kogler GF, Solomonidis SE, Paul JP. Biomechanics of longitudinal arch support mechanisms in foot orthoses and their effect on plantar aponeurosis strain. Clin Biomech (Bristol, Avon). 11(5):243–52, 1996.

150. Fleischer AE, Albright RH, Crews RT, Kelil T, Wrobel JS. Prognostic value of diagnostic sonography in patients with plantar fasciitis. J Ultrasound Med. 34(10):1729–35, 2015.

151. Cheung RT, Chung RC, Ng GY. Efficacies of different external controls for excessive foot pronation: a meta-analysis. Br J Sports Med. 45(9):743–51, 2011.

152. Abd El Salam MD, Abd Elharz YN. Low-Dye taping versus medial arch support in managing pain and pain-related disability in patients with plantar fasciitis. Foot Ankle Spec. 4(2):86–91, 2011.

153. Yucel U, Kucuksen HT, Anliacik E, Ozbek O, Salli A, Ugurlu H. Full-length silicone insoles versus ultrasound-guided corticosteroid injection in the management of plantar fasciitis: a randomized clinical trial. Prosthet Orthot Int. 37(6):471–6, 2013.

154. Lin SC, Chen CP, Tang SF, Wong AM, Hsieh JH, Chen WP. Changes in windlass effect in response to different shoe and insole designs during walking. Gait Posture. 37(2):235–41, 2013.

155. Karagounis P, Tsironi M, Prionas G, Tsiganos G, Baltopoulos P. Treatment of plantar fasciitis in recreational athletes: two different therapeutic protocols. Foot Ankle Spec. 4(4):226–34, 2011.

156. DiGiovanni BF, Nawoczenski DA, Lintal ME, Moore EA, Murray JC, Wilding GE, Baumhauer JF. Tissue-specific plantar fascia-stretching exercise enhances outcomes in patients with chronic heel pain: A prospective, randomized study. J Bone Joint Surg Am. 85-A(7):1270–7, 2003.

157. Wrobel JS, Fleischer AE, Matzkin-Bridger J, Fascione J, Crews RT, Bruning N, Jarrett B. Physical examination variables predict response to conservative treatment of nonchronic plantar fasciitis: secondary analysis of a randomized, placebo-controlled footwear study. PM R. 8(5):436–44, 2016.

158. Radford JA, Landorf KB, Buchbinder R, Cook C. Effectiveness of calf muscle stretching for the short-term treatment of plantar heel pain: a randomized trial. BMC Musculoskelet Disord. 19(8):36, 2007.

159. Barry LD, Barry AN, Chen Y. A retrospective study of standing gastrocnemius-soleus stretching versus night splinting in the treatment of plantar fasciitis. J Foot Ankle Surg. 41(4):221–7, 2002.

160. Brook J, Dauphinee DM, Korpinen J, Rawe IM. Pulsed radiofrequency electromagnetic field therapy: a potential novel treatment of plantar fasciitis. J Foot Ankle Surg. 51(3):312–6, 2012.

161. Lou J, Wang S, Liu S, Xing G. Effectiveness of extracorporeal shock wave therapy without local anesthesia in patients with recalcitrant plantar fasciitis: a meta-analysis of randomized controlled trials. Am J Phys Med Rehabil. 2016. (Epub ahead of print.)

162. Lizis P. Comparison between real and placebo extracorporeal shockwave therapy for the treatment of chronic plantar fasciitis in males. Iran J Public Health. 44(8):1150–2, 2015.

163. Chew KT, Leong D, Lin CY, Lim KK, Tan B. Comparison of autologous conditioned plasma injection, extracorporeal shockwave therapy, and conventional treatment for plantar fasciitis: a randomized trial. PR R. 5(12):1035–43, 2013.

164. Wang CY, Wang FS, Yang KD, Weng LH, Ko JY. Long-term results of extracorporeal shockwave treatment for plantar fasciitis. Am J Sports Med. 34(4):592–6, 2006.

165. Hammer DS, Rupp S, Kreutz A, Pape D, Kohn D, Seil R. Extracorporeal shockwave therapy (ESWT) in patients with chronic proximal plantar fasciitis. Foot Ankle Int. 23(4):309–13, 2002.

166. Othman AM, Ragab EM. Endoscopic plantar fasciotomy versus extra-corporeal shock wave therapy for treatment of chronic plantar fasciitis. Arch Orthop Trauma Surg. 130(11):1343–7, 2010.

167. Macias DM, Coughlin MJ, Zhang K, Stevens FR, Jastifer JR, Doty JF. Low-level laser therapy at 635 nm for treatment of chronic plantar fasciitis: a placebo-controlled, randomized study. J Foot Ankle Surg. 54(5):768–72, 2015.

168. Winemiller MH, Billow RG, Laskowski ER, Harmsen WS. Effect of magnetic vs sham-magnetic insoles on plantar heel pain: a randomized controlled trial. JAMA. 290(11):1474–8, 2003.

169. Weintraub MI. Magnets for patients with heel pain. JAMA. 291(1):43–4, 2004.

170. Sorensen MD, Hyer CH, Philibin TM. Percutaneous bipolar radiofrequency microdebridement for recalcitrant proximal plantar fasciosis. J Foot Ankle Surg. 50(2):165–70, 2011.

171. Davies MS, Weiss GA, Saxby TS. Plantar fasciitis: how successful is surgical intervention? Foot Ankle Int. 20(12):803–7, 1999.

172. Landsman AS, Catanese DJ, Wiener SN, Richie DH, Hanft JR. A prospective, randomized, double-blinded study with crossover to determine the efficacy of radio-frequency nerve ablation for the treatment of heel pain. J Am Podiatr Med Assoc. 103(1):8–15, 2013.

173. Krken HY, Ayanoglu S, Akmaz I, Erler K, Kiral A. Prospective study of percutaneous radiofrequency nerve ablation for chronic plantar fasciitis. Foot Ankle Int. 35(2):95–103, 2014.

174. Sorensen MD, Hyer CH, Philibin TM. Percutaneous bipolar radiofrequency microdebridement for recalcitrant proximal plantar fasciosis. J Foot Ankle Surg. 50(2):165–70, 2011.

175. Weil L Jr., Glover JP, Weil LS Sr. A new minimally invasive technique for treatment of plantar fasciosis using bipolar radiofrequency: a prospective analysis. Foot Ankle Spec. 1(1):13–18, 2008.

176. Micke O, Seegnenschmiedt MH, Mucke R, de Vries A, Schafer U, Willich N. Plantar fasciitis and radiotherapy. Clinical and radiobiological treatment results. Orthopade. 34(6):579–91, 2005.

177. Arslan A, Koca TT, Utkan A, Sevimli R, Akel J. Treatment of chronic plantar heel pain with radiofrequency neural ablation of the first branch of the lateral plantar nerve and medical calcaneal nerve branches. J Foot Ankle Surg. 55(4):767–71, 2016.

178. Hormozi J, Lee S, Hong DK. Minimal invasive percutaneous bipolar radiofrequency for plantar fasciotomy: a retrospective study. J Foot Ankle Surg. 50(3):283–6, 2011.

179. Costantino C, Vulpiani MC, Romiti D, Vetrano M, Saraceni VM. Cryoultrasound therapy in the treatment of chronic plantar fasciitis with heel spurs. A randomized controlled clinical study. Eur J Phys Rehabil Med. 50(1):39–47, 2014.

180. Cavazos GJ, Khan KH, D'Antoni AV, Harkless LB, Lopez D. Cryosurgery for the treatment of heel pain. Foot Ankle Int. 30(6):500–5, 2009.

181. Liang J, Yang Y, Yu G, Niu W, Wang Y. Deformation and stress distribution of the human foot after plantar ligaments release: a cadaver study and finite element analysis. Sci China Life Sci. 54(3):267–71, 2011.

182. Tao K, Ji WT, Wang DM, Wang CT, Wang X. Relative contributions of plantar fascia and ligaments on the arch static stability: a finite element study. Biomed Tech (Berl). 55(5):265–71, 2010.

183. Iaquinto JM, Wayne JS. Computational model of the lower leg and foot/ankle complex: application to arch stability. J Biomech Eng. 132(2):021009, 2010.

184. Gefen A. Stress analysis of the standing foot following surgical plantar fascia release. J Biomech. 35(5):629–37, 2002.

185. Saxena A, Fournier M, Gerdesmeyer L, Gollwitzer H. Comparison between extracorporeal shockwave therapy, placebo ESWT and endoscopic plantar fasciotomy for the treatment of chronic plantar heel pain in the athlete. Muscles Ligaments Tendons J. 2(4):312–6, 2013.

186. Fallat LM, Cox JT, Chahal R, Morrison P, Kish J. A retrospective comparison of percutaneous plantar fasciotomy and open plantar fasciotomy with heel spur resection. J Foot Ankle Surg. 52(3):288–90, 2013.

187. Radwan YA, Mansour AM, Badawy WS. Resistant plantar fasciotomy: shock wave versus endoscopic plantar fascial release. Int Orthop. 36(10):2147–32, 2012.

188. Bader L, Park K, Gu Y, O'Malley MJ. Functional outcome of endoscopic plantar fasciotomy. Foot Ankle Int. 33(1):37–43, 2012.

189. Hogan KA, Webb D, Shereff M. Endoscopic plantar fascia release. Foot Ankle Int. 25(12):875–81, 2004.

190. Brugh AM, Fallat LM, Savoy-Moore RT. Lateral column symptomatology following plantar fascial release: a prospective study. J Foot Ankle Surg. 41(6):365–71, 2002.

191. Cheung JT, An KN, Zhang M. Consequences of partial and total plantar fascia release: a finite element study. Foot Ankle Int. 27(2):125–32, 2006.

192. Yu JS, Spigos D, Tomczak R. Foot pain after a plantar fasciotomy: an MR analysis to determine potential causes. J Comput Assist Tomogr. 23(5):707–12, 1999.

193. Pontious J, Flanigan KP, Hillstrom HJ. Role of the plantar fascia in digital stabilization: A case report. J Am Podiatr Med Assoc. 86(1):43–7, 1996.

194. Sammarco GJ, Idusuyi OB. Stress fracture of the base of the third metatarsal after an endoscopic plantar fasciotomy: a case report. Foot Ankle Int. 19(3):157–9, 1998.

195. Yu JS, Spigos D, Tomczak R. Foot pain after a plantar fasciotomy: an MR analysis to determine potential causes. J Comput Assist Tomogr. 23(5):707–12, 1999.

196. Sharkey NA, Donahue SW, Ferris L. Biomechanical consequences of plantar fascial release or rupture during gait. Part II: alterations in forefoot loading. Foot Ankle Int. 20(2):86–96, 1999.

197. Murphy GA, Pneumaticos SG, Kamaric E, Noble PC, Trevino SG, Baxter DE. Biomechanical consequences of sequential plantar fascial release. Foot Ankle Int. 19(3):149–52, 1998.

198. Smith S, Tinley P, Gilheany M, Grills B, Kingsford A. The inferior calcaneal spur—Anatomical and histological considerations. The Foot. 17(1): 25–31, 2007.

199. Kirkpatrick J, Yassaie O, Mirjalili SA. The plantar calcaneal spur: a review of anatomy, histology, etiology and key associations. J Anat. Jun;230(6):743–751, 2017.

200. Li J, Muehleman C. Anatomic relationship of heel spur to surrounding soft tissues: greater variability than previously reported. Clin Anat. 20(8):950–5, 2007.

201. Perry J. Anatomy and biomechanics of the hindfoot. Clin Orthop Relat Res. 177:9–15, 1983.

202. Ehrmann C, Majer M, Mengiardi B, Pfirrmann CW, Sutter R. Calcaneal attachment of the plantar fascia: MR findings in asymptomatic volunteers. Radiology. 272(3):807–14, 2014.

203. Ahmad J, Karim A, Daniel JN. Relationship and Classification of Plantar Heel Spurs in Patients with Plantar Fasciitis. Foot Ankle Int. Sep;37(9):994–1000, 2016.

204. Fallat LM, Cox JT, Chahal R, Morrison P, Kish J. A retrospective comparison of percutaneous plantar fasciotomy and open plantar fasciotomy with heel spur resection. J Foot Ankle Surg. 2013 May-Jun;52(3):288–90.

205. Apostol-Gonzalez S, Herrera J, Herrera I. Calcaneus fracture as a complication of the percutaneous treatment of plantar fasciitis: Case report. Acta Ortop Mex. 28(2):134–6, 2014.

206. Kumai T, Benjamin M. Heel spur formation and the subcalcaneal enthesis of the plantar fascia. J Rheumatol. 29(9):1957–64, 2002.

207. Osborne HR, Breidahl WH, Allison GT. Critical differences in lateral X-rays with and without a diagnosis of plantar fasciitis. J Sci Med Sport. 9(3):231–7, 2006.

208. Jarde O, Diebold P, Havet E, Boulu G, Vernois J. Degenerative lesions of the plantar fascia: surgical treatment by fasciectomy and excision of the heel spur: A report of 38 cases. Acta Orthop Belg. 69(3):267–74, 2003.

209. Monteagudo M, Maceira E, Garcia-Virto V, Canosa R. Chronic plantar fasciitis: plantar fasciotomy versus gastrocnemius recession. Int Orthop. 37(9):1845–50, 2013.

210. Miyamoto W, Takao M, Uchino Y. Calcaneal osteotomy for the treatment of plantar fasciitis. Arch Orthop Trauma Surg. 130(2):151–4, 2010.

211. Horton GA, Myerson MS, Parks BG, Park YW. Effect of calcaneal osteotomy and lateral column lengthening on the plantar fascia: a biomechanical investigation. Foot Ankle Int. 19(6):370–3, 1998.

Chapter 13

212. Graham ME, Jawrani NT, Goel VK. Evaluating plantar fascia strain in hyperpronating cadaveric feet following an extra-osseous talotarsal stabilization procedure. J Foot Ankle Surg. 50(6):682–6, 2011.

213. Xu Y, Li SC, Xu SY. Calcaneal Z lengthening osteotomy combined with subtalar arthroereisis for severe adolescent flexible flatfoot reconstruction. Foot Ankle Int. 37(11):1225–31, 2016.

214. Steber S, Kolodziej L. Analysis of radiographic outcomes comparing foot orthosis to extra-osseous talotarsal stabilization in the treatment of recurrent talotarsal joint dislocation. J Min Inv Orthop. 1:1–11, 2015.

215. Graham, ME. Congenital talotarsal joint displacement and pes planovalgus. Clin Podiatr Med Surg. 30:567–81, 2013.

216. Bresnahan PJ, Chariton JT, Vedpathak A. Extra-osseous talotarsal stabilization using HyProCure®: preliminary clinical outcomes of a prospective case series. J Foot Ankle Surg. 52(2):195–202, 2013.

217. Fitzgerald RH, Vedpathak A. Plantar pressure distribution in a hyperpronated foot before and after intervention with an extra-osseous talotarsal stabilization device—a retrospective study. J Foot Ankle Surg. 52(4):432–43, 2013.

218. Navi B, Theivendran K, Prem H. Computed tomography review of tarsal canal anatomy with reference to the fitting of sinus tarsi implants in the tarsal canal. J Foot Ankle Surg. 52(6):714–6, 2013.

219. Graham ME, Jawrani NT. Extra-osseous stabilization devices: a new classification system. J Foot Ankle Surg. 51(5):613–9, 2012.

220. Graham ME, Jawrani, NT, Chikka A. Extra-osseous talotarsal stabilization using HyProCure® in adults: a 5-year retrospective follow-up. J Foot Ankle Surg. 51(1):23–9, 2012.

221. Graham ME, Jawrani NT, Chikka A, Rogers RJ. Surgical treatment of hyperpronation using an extra-osseous talotarsal stabilization device: radiographic outcomes in adult patients. J Foot Ankle Surg. 51(5):548–55, 2012.

222. Graham ME, Jawrani NT, Chikka A. Radiographic evaluation of navicular position in the sagittal plane—correction following an extra-osseous talotarsal stabilization procedure. J Foot Ankle Surg. 50(5):551–7, 2011.

223. Graham ME, Jawrani NT, Goel VK. Effect of extra-osseous talotarsal stabilization on posterior tibial tendon strain in hyperpronating feet. J Foot Ankle Surg. 50(6):676–81, 2011.

224. Graham ME, Parikh R, Goel V, Mhatre D, Matyas A. Stabilization of joint forces of the subtalar complex via HyProCure sinus tarsi stent. J Am Podiatr Med Assoc. 101(5):390–9, 2011.

225. Graham ME. Talotarsal joint displacement—diagnosis and stabilization options. Foot Ankle Quarterly. 23(4):165–179, 2012.

226. Graham ME, Jawrani NT, Goel VK. Evaluating plantar fascia strain in hyperpronating cadaveric feet following an extra-osseous talotarsal stabilization procedure. J Foot Ankle Surg. 50(6):682–6, 2011.

227. Graham ME, Jawrani NT, Goel VK. Effect of extra-osseous talotarsal stabilization on posterior tibial nerve strain in hyperpronating feet: a cadaveric evaluation. J Foot Ankle Surg. 50(6):672–5, 2011.

228. Graham ME, Jawrani NT, Goel VK. The effect of HyProCure® on tarsal tunnel compartment pressures in hyperpronating feet. J Foot Ankle Surg. 50(1):44–9, 2011.

About the Author

Michael E. Graham, DPM, FACFAS, FAENS, FAAFAS, FACFAP
Dr. Michael E. Graham is board-certified by the American Board of Foot and Ankle Surgery, a Fellow of the American College of Foot and Ankle Surgeons, a Fellow of the Association of Extremity Nerve Surgeons, a Fellow of the Academy of Ambulatory Foot and Ankle Surgeons, and a Fellow of the American College of Foot and Ankle Pediatrics. He is the founder and director of the Graham International Implant Institute, as well as CEO and founder of GraMedica. Dr. Graham is an internationally renowned speaker and has published many scientific articles in leading peer-reviewed medical journals. He is licensed to practice podiatric medicine and surgery in the state of Michigan. Dr. Graham has been named Podiatry Management VIP among podiatrists. He serves on the Board of Visitors of Temple University School of Podiatric Medicine and is a professor at the Academy of Ambulatory Foot and Ankle Surgery.

His interest in the foot and ankle began at the age of seven, and he gained early acceptance into the Temple University School of Podiatric Medicine. After graduating with his doctorate, he completed his surgical residency at Kern Hospital for Special Surgery in Warren, Michigan. He was very successful in private practice, with more than fifteen years of clinical experience.

Dr. Graham is also the inventor of the HyProCure sinus tarsi implant. This unique medical device, which received FDA clearance in 2004, is inserted into a naturally occurring space between the ankle-bone and heel bone to instantly realign the hindfoot. HyProCure is now available in more than seventy countries.

CPSIA information can be obtained
at www.ICGtesting.com
Printed in the USA
FFHW022317120919
54959739-60662FF